THE LITTLE ENCYCLOPEDIA
OF HERBAL MEDICINE

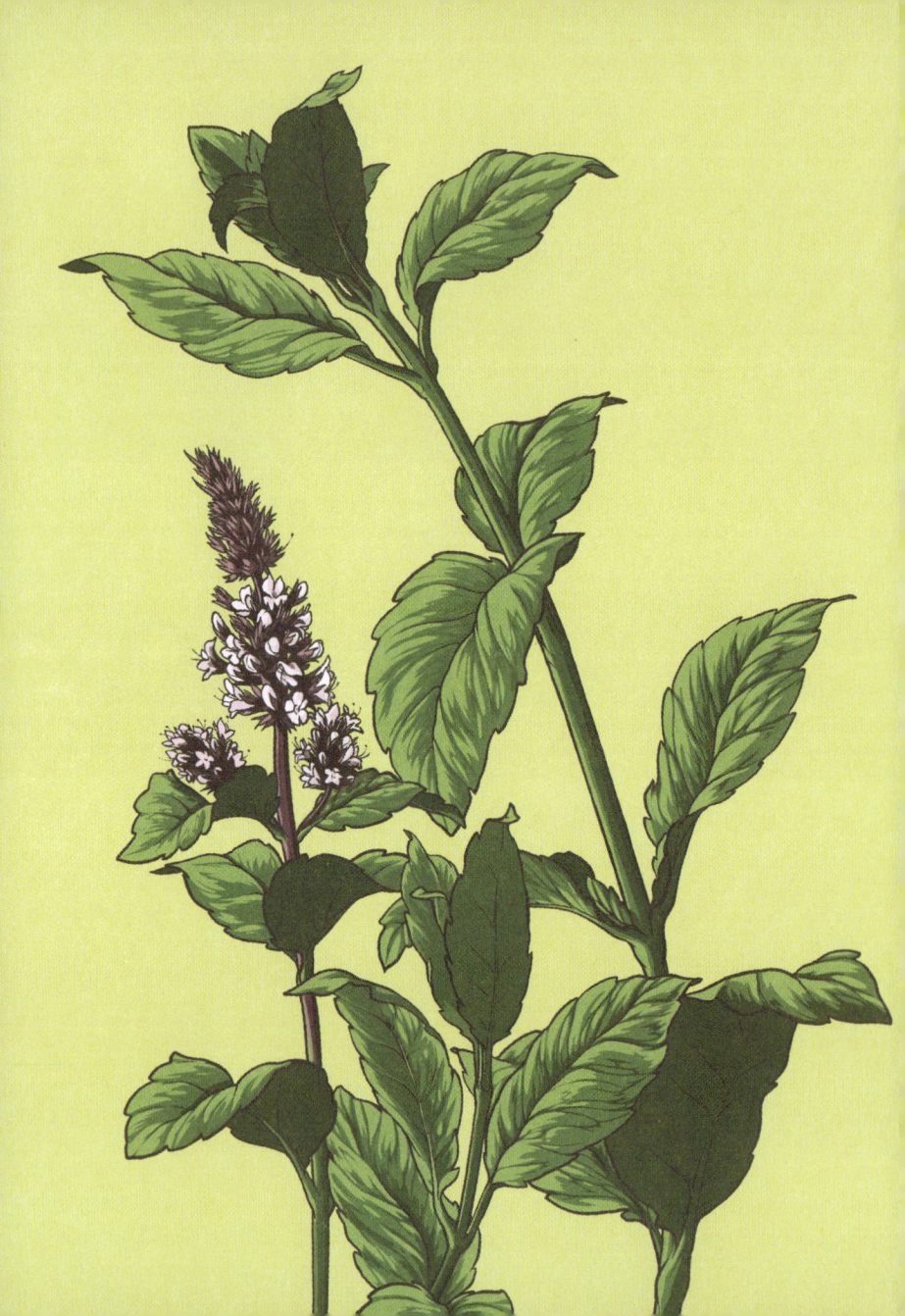

THE

LITTLE ENCYCLOPEDIA

OF

Herbal
Medicine

100 Common Remedies for
Everyday Ailments

ANGELA RENZETTI, LAc, EAMP, RH

Illustrations by Amanda Key

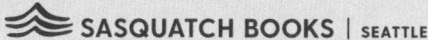
SASQUATCH BOOKS | SEATTLE

HEALTH DISCLAIMER

This book is for educational purposes only and does not replace professional medical advice, diagnosis, or treatment. Always consult your healthcare provider before using herbal remedies, especially if you have a medical condition, take prescription medications, are pregnant or nursing, or are treating a child.

Herbs can interact with medications and reduce or change their efficacy. "Natural" doesn't mean safe for everyone. Start with small amounts, follow dosages carefully, and discontinue use if adverse reactions occur. For serious symptoms, seek immediate medical attention.

The statements in this book have not been evaluated by the US Food and Drug Administration. These remedies are not intended to diagnose, treat, cure, or prevent any disease.

Children, elderly individuals, and those with compromised immune systems should use extra caution. Some herbs are inappropriate during pregnancy or breastfeeding. When foraging, ensure proper plant identification—when in doubt, purchase from reputable suppliers.

The author and publisher disclaim liability from the use of information in this book. You are responsible for your own health decisions. This book is educational—not a replacement for professional medical care. Work with your healthcare provider to safely integrate herbal remedies into your wellness routine.

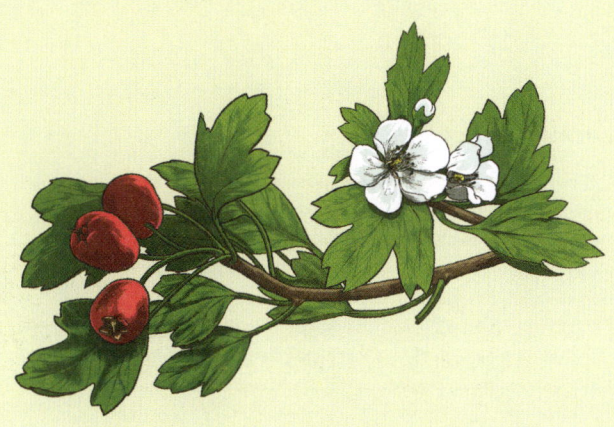

This book is dedicated to anyone looking to connect more with plants. Nature calls you back home.

To all my patients, students, and teachers over the years, thank you.

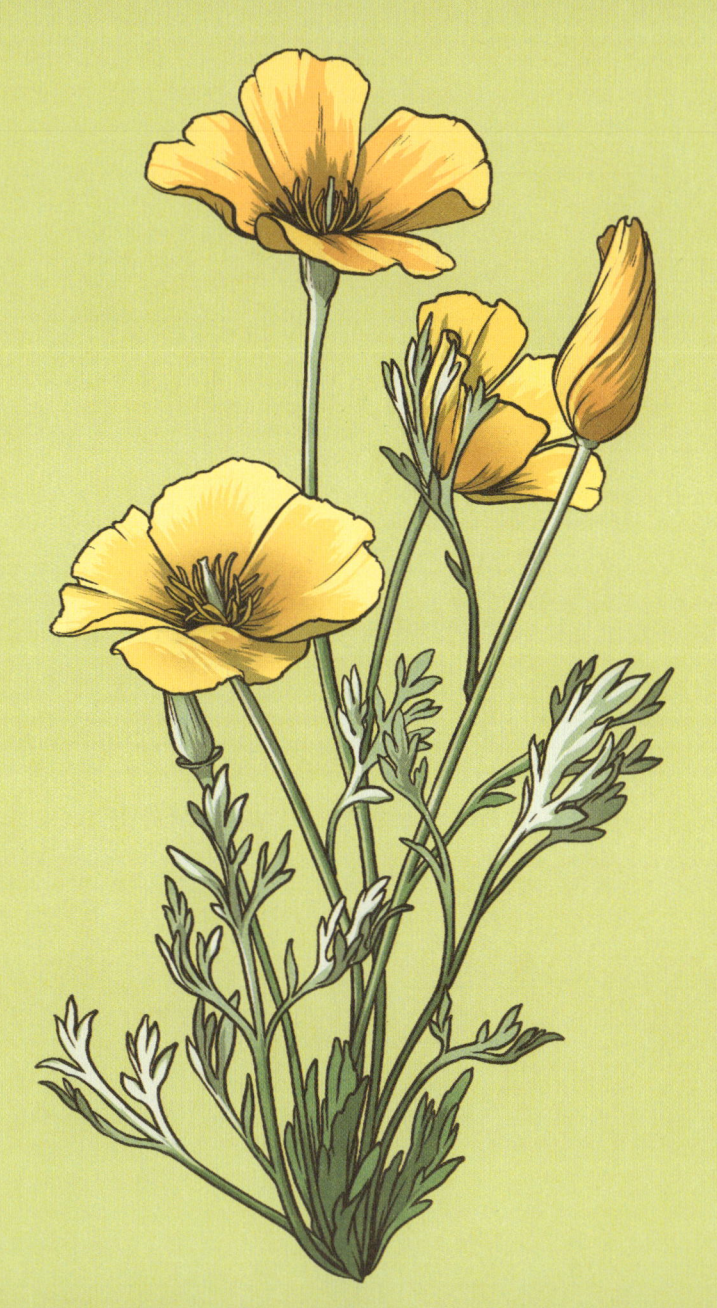

Contents

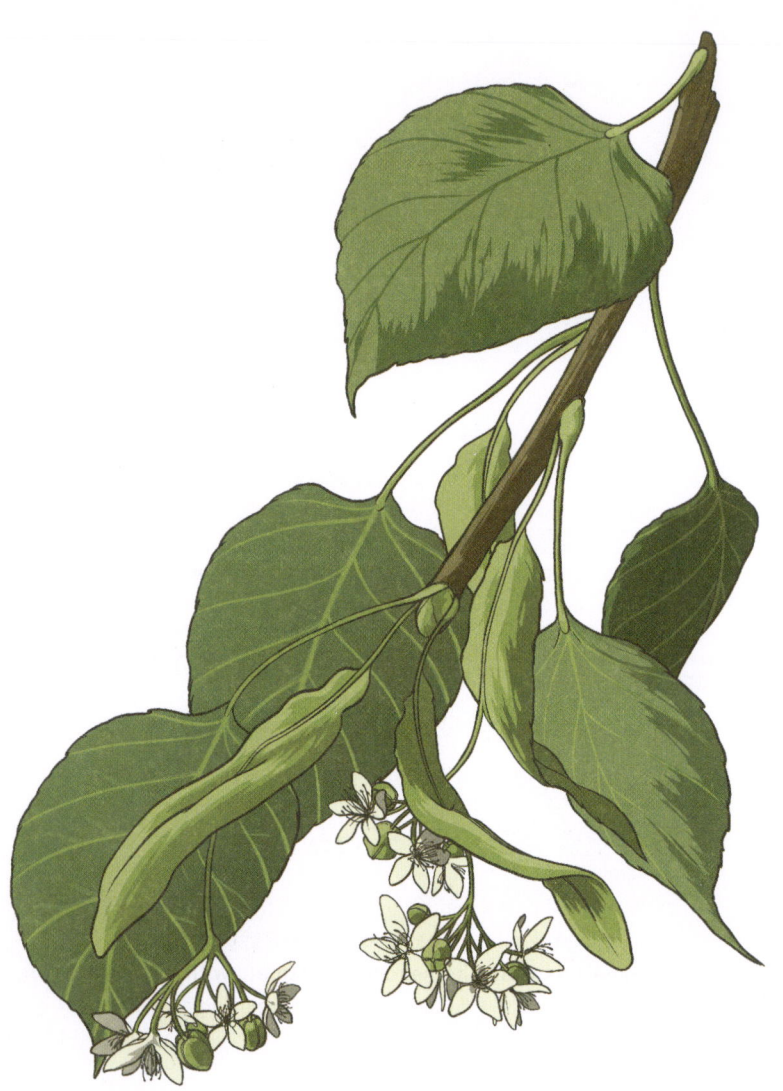

Introduction

I began studying herbal medicine when I moved back to Seattle from China in 2011. I'd been living in Sichuan, working as a Chinese–English translator and singing in a band. During my years there, I'd gotten sick several times and discovered the power of traditional remedies.

Below my Chengdu courtyard stretched a row of Chinese medicine doctors and herb dispensaries. My Mandarin was good, but my Sichuanese was nonexistent, making it challenging to communicate when I needed help with a cold or stomachache. The herbalist would examine my tongue, take my pulse, and then gather herbs from countless drawers, scooping them into a paper bag—it felt like stepping back in time. I'd wobble home to my apartment with the earthy, bitter, pungent herbs and prepare them using a traditional method called a decoction (which we'll explore more in this book). When I had a head cold, the healing often began as soon as the herbs started to cook—the aromatic vapors filled my apartment, and I could feel my sinuses opening even before taking a sip. And after just the first cup of the decoction, I would often feel my headache ease, my body relax, and my symptoms begin to lift, feeling better immediately. What was this magic? Growing up on over-the-counter drugs and processed foods, natural medicine was foreign to me. When I befriended Israeli students studying acupuncture in Chengdu, my fascination with Traditional Chinese Medicine truly began.

Two years later I moved home to Seattle, planning to attend acupuncture school. But life rarely follows our plans. That summer severe reverse culture shock left me deeply depressed. One afternoon, wandering through Ballard, I discovered Dandelion Botanical Company advertising fall herbalism classes that combined local and Chinese herbs. This became my entry point—studying Chinese, Ayurvedic, and Western herbs with K. P. Khalsa at the International Integrative Educational Institute. Reconnecting with the Pacific Northwest landscape, and learning about plants I'd grown up with but never understood, proved deeply healing. My connection with nature restored my mind and spirit. Two years later I finally started acupuncture school.

During school I worked at Rainbow Natural Remedies, a Seattle wellness store with an incredible apothecary. Day after day customers arrived seeking remedies but lacking basic herbal knowledge. They didn't know what a tincture was or how to prepare tea. Recognizing this need, I began teaching beginner herbalism classes, continuing for years to help people understand their options.

In my experience with herbal remedy books, I've noticed two persistent problems: poor indexing that makes finding specific remedies difficult and authors who lack the clinical experience to verify what actually works. Having run a clinic, taught countless students, and maintained my love of research, I've created something different—a book organized alphabetically by ailment, not by herb, so you can quickly find exactly what you need.

I hope this book introduces you to plant allies that make your life better. Nature calls you back home.

—Angela

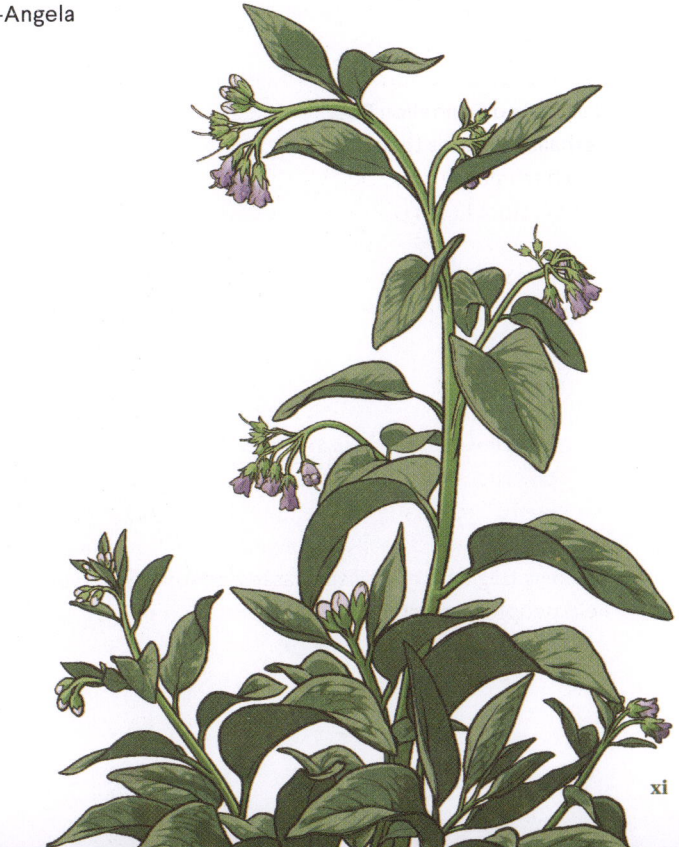

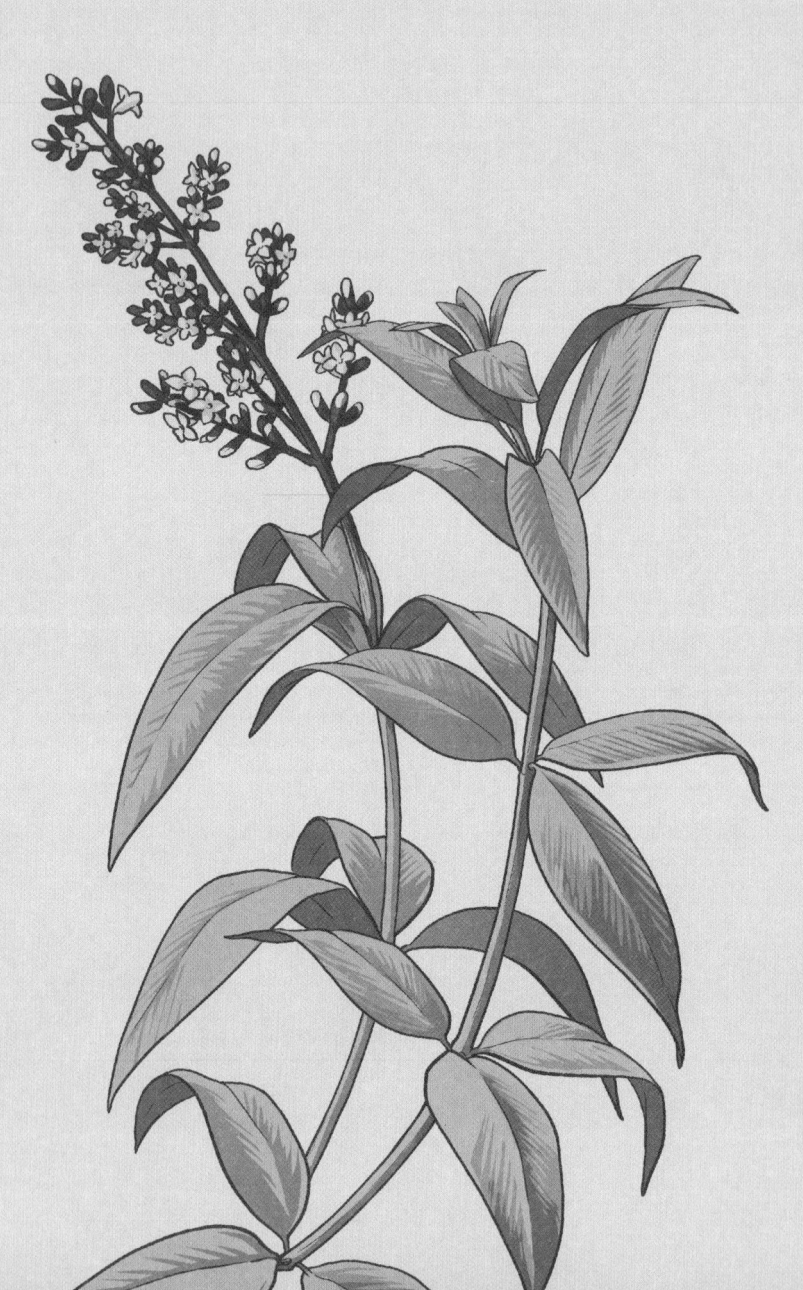

Herbal Remedies and How to Use Them

H

erbal medicine is a lifelong journey. After fourteen years of study and practice, I'm still discovering new things. This book distills my experience as a clinical and folk herbalist into a practical guide for treating everyday ailments at home with proven plant allies.

Part I is essential foundational knowledge—please don't skip it. When you encounter questions in later sections, return here for clarity.

BRIEF HISTORY OF HERBAL MEDICINE

Herbs are simply plants, and humans have used them throughout their existence—for food, medicine, bathing, building, spiritual practices, and more. Even today, when people don't realize that they're using herbs, intuition often guides them. The spices in your kitchen, the plants in your bathroom, the flowers given for luck—all carry centuries of traditional use. Those kitchen aromatics, for instance, weren't originally valued just for their flavor but for their antibacterial properties.

When I began studying herbal medicine, I didn't understand the scope of its usage throughout the world. In the United States, we often focus on established systems: Traditional Chinese Medicine, Western European herbalism, homeopathy, and Ayurveda. Each has distinct methods for diagnosing illness and formulating remedies. Yet every culture has its own native herbalism—folk medicine passed down through generations. In remote villages around the world, local herbalists know which plants can treat common ailments.

Consider how different systems approach a simple cough. In my Chinese medicine practice, I assess the patient's health history, cough quality, illness duration, and other factors. My diagnosis recommends a formula combining multiple complementary herbs, addressing both the primary complaint and constitutional needs. When the patient calls a week later with resolved symptoms but lingering weakness, we adjust the formula to support recovery. Western herbalism follows a similar individualized approach.

Folk herbalism, which many recipes in this book represent, takes a simpler path. You might already use garden herbs or kitchen ingredients to treat a symptom—rosemary steam for congestion, sage tea for a sore throat. Perhaps your grandmother made onion syrup whenever someone in the family was sick. These practitioners may lack formal training, but they understand which plants help specific conditions.

After years of clinical practice, I've learned that no system is superior—each serves different needs effectively.

BUYING HERBS

Finding quality herbs depends on your location, but several reliable sources exist.

Start with local herbal apothecaries if available. These shops offer dried herbs, prepared remedies, and knowledgeable staff. Natural food stores often stock bulk herbs—though marketed for cooking, many double as medicine. Farmers' markets frequently feature vendors growing medicinal plants.

When buying locally isn't possible, reputable online suppliers deliver quality herbs nationwide. Mountain Rose Herbs and Starwest Botanicals offer extensive selections. Smaller operations such as High Garden in Nashville provide carefully sourced or wildcrafted herbs. Some herbalists sell directly from their farms.

Regardless of the source, prioritize quality. Ask about organic certification, wildcrafting practices, and freshness. Good suppliers will gladly share this information.

GROWING HERBS

Growing medicinal plants connects you directly with your remedies. Consider what herbs will be most useful and then think about how you could grow them at home. Start simple—even a sunny windowsill can support a few pots.

Culinary herbs such as lavender, rosemary, thyme, and sage are quite versatile, and they tolerate container growing. When you cut back a little, they'll often regenerate after harvesting. Other herbs such as lemon balm or mint thrive in pots, producing abundant leaves. You can snip them off fresh or cut off stems and make little bundles to hang and dry from the ceiling or wall.

Consider your health needs when selecting plants. For example, if you are experiencing perimenopause, motherwort could be a great herb to grow on your patio. Then plan ahead. That motherwort tincture made today might prove invaluable later. Some herbs are also difficult to grow; roots usually need a long time, sometimes one to three years, to yield medicine. Consider focusing on aerial parts (leaves and flowers), which are much easier to grow and are often perennial.

Container gardens suit most medicinal herbs, and many may come back the following year if tended properly. Some plants such as roses are shrublike and need more space. Even if you never harvest them, watching plants grow deepens your understanding of their medicine, which can be healing in and of itself. Notice their preferred conditions, companion plants, and seasonal changes. This observation teaches what no book can capture.

Local nurseries increasingly stock medicinal plants. Staff can recommend varieties suited to your climate and space.

MAKING HERBAL MEDICINES

Creating your own remedies transforms herbs into medicine, but it may take practice. My first attempts failed spectacularly—moldy tinctures, rancid oils, and forgotten jars. Through these mistakes, I learned that success requires attention to cleanliness and process.

This book primarily uses folk methods—simpler than professional preparations but effective. When I specify "parts," I'm describing a versatile measurement that allows you to scale recipes. Start with 1 tablespoon as 1 part for small batches. Once you've tested a recipe, scale up using 1 ounce as 1 part.

Cleanliness prevents contamination. Sterilize jars, sanitize work surfaces, and wash your hands thoroughly. This matters most for oils and salves, which spoil easily. Teas and tinctures resist contamination better due to the use of hot water and alcohol.

MAKING TEA (INFUSIONS & DECOCTIONS)

Infusions (Hot & Cold)

Infusions extract medicine from delicate parts of the plant, such as flowers and leaves, by steeping the dried herbs in hot or cold water. While fresh plants can be used, all recipes in this book call for dried herbs.

HOT INFUSIONS: A hot infusion, or what we typically call "making tea," uses 1 heaping tablespoon of herb per cup of water. Place herbs in a vessel (teapot, cup with strainer, or French press), pour boiling water over them, and steep for 15 to 30 minutes. Mild herbs like milky oats or horsetail can steep for hours. When creating your own blends, remember that some herbs turn bitter quickly while others need longer steeping times. Start with 10 to 15 minutes and increase if the remedy isn't too bitter.

COLD INFUSIONS: Cold infusions work best for plants that have mucilage, a therapeutic gooey substance made of proteins and polysaccharides. Marshmallow root and nettle are prime examples.

To make a cold infusion, use 1 heaping tablespoon of herb per cup of cool water. Place the herbs in your vessel, pour water over the herbs, stir or shake, and then steep on the counter overnight or refrigerate for at least 4 hours. Strain and serve.

> *Tip:* When drinking multiple cups daily, prep a large batch. Make a quart in a French press in the morning, using 4 tablespoons herb to 1 quart water. By the time you're ready to leave, it's cool enough to transfer to a jar or thermos for work.

Decoctions

Decoctions extract medicine from tougher parts of the plant—berries, twigs, roots, mushrooms, and seeds—that need extended heating.

Place the herbs in a small saucepan and cover with water. Heat slowly without boiling, and simmer for 15 to 30 minutes. Use 1 teaspoon to 1 tablespoon per cup of water (add extra water to account for evaporation). Strain and serve.

Both infusions and decoctions will last in the refrigerator for about 3 days.

TINCTURES & LINIMENTS

Tinctures are alcohol-based extracts for internal use, while liniments are for external application. Alcohol efficiently extracts medicinal components and preserves them longer than water. While vinegar, wine, or vegetable glycerin (glycerin preparations are called glycerites) can also be used, this book uses alcohol-based tinctures.

Folk Tinctures Versus Weight-to-Volume Method

This book uses the folk method, which is simpler than the precise weight-to-volume calculations used professionally. While folk tinctures don't provide exact milligram dosages, they're effective for home use. For detailed information on precise methods, consult James Green's *The Herbal Medicine Maker's Handbook: A Home Manual* or Richo Cech's *Making Plant Medicine.*

Folk Tincture Method

Fill a jar halfway with dried herbs (¾ full for fresh plants). Cover completely with alcohol (80 to 100 proof vodka or brandy work well). Lid and shake. Check after a few hours—if the herbs have risen above the alcohol line, add more. Label with the herb name and date. Store in a cool, dark place and shake daily to ensure good extraction. After 4 weeks, strain through a cheesecloth-lined mesh strainer into a Pyrex container. Squeeze the cloth to extract the liquid. Transfer to amber dropper bottles or clean jars.

Mixing Premade Tinctures

If you prefer buying tinctures (Herb Pharm is widely available), you can mix them yourself. For each "part" in a recipe, use 1 dropperful or teaspoon. Combine in a separate container and dose as needed. Try individual herbs first to learn how your body responds to each one.

Note: Some recipes include honey (typically ¾ alcohol and ¼ honey). These sweetened tinctures are often called elixirs or cordials.

SYRUPS

Syrups preserve herbal decoctions with sugar. While cane sugar works best, mixing honey and brandy reduces sugar content and maintains preservation.

GENERAL METHOD: Simmer ½ to 1 cup of dried herb in 1 quart of water for 45 to 60 minutes, reducing the liquid by ¼ to ⅓. Place a strainer on top of a measuring cup and strain the liquid from the pan. Add equal parts sugar to liquid (1 cup liquid = 1 cup sugar).

For less sugar, substitute ¾ cup honey plus ¼ cup brandy per cup of sugar needed. Less sugar means a shorter shelf life.

OILS

Herbal oil can be made in several ways. Herb-to-oil ratios vary by method:

SOLAR INFUSION: Fill your jar ¾ full with herb, then cover with oil.

DOUBLE BOILER/ALCOHOL-INTERMEDIARY METHOD: 1 cup whole herb (¼ to ½ cup powdered) per 1 to 1.5 cups oil

Olive oil is most commonly used, but sesame, grapeseed, almond, and apricot oils work well. Jojoba and castor oils are generally too thick.

Solar-Infused Oils

Cover the herbs with oil in a jar. Place the jar in a sunny, warm spot for about 3 weeks, shaking gently daily. Strain the oil through a cheesecloth and wring out the herbs thoroughly. For stronger oil, repeat with fresh herbs for 2 more weeks. Store in a cool, dark place for up to 2 years.

Double-Boiler Method

Heat the herbs and oil in a double boiler at a low simmer for 1 to 2 hours, monitoring to prevent overheating or burning. You can do this in a slow cooker as well, which you can leave for 3 to 4 hours. Strain the oil through a cheesecloth and then wring it thoroughly.

Alcohol-Intermediary Method (My Favorite)

Blend your herbs on high in a blender until they are nearly a powder. Transfer to a bowl and moisten with 1 to 2 teaspoons of alcohol (80 to 100 proof vodka works well), mashing to eliminate clumps. Let it sit for 30 minutes. Then add the herbs back into the blender with your oil and blend for 5 to 10 minutes. Pause if your blender overheats. Pour this mixture into a jar, let it sit for 2 weeks, and then strain through a muslin cloth for a potent oil.

SALVES

You can transform herbal oil into portable medicine with beeswax (or candelilla wax for a vegan option).

RATIO: 4 ounces of oil to 2 tablespoons of beeswax pastilles. More beeswax creates a firmer salve. Firmness helps the salve be transportable, but if you plan to mostly keep it at home under cool conditions, you can use less beeswax.

Heat the oil in a double boiler without boiling. Add beeswax, stirring with a chopstick until melted. Pour immediately into containers and let it harden overnight before lidding.

Tip: If you don't have a double boiler, create a makeshift version by setting a glass jar inside a saucepan filled with a couple inches of water. To avoid the glass breaking, place a washcloth inside. You can also place a stainless-steel topper in the saucepan. Be sure the water and oil don't mix, as it'll make the mixture go rancid faster.

BATHS & SOAKS

FOOT OR HAND SOAKS: Steep 1 cup of dried herb in ½ gallon of hot water for 30 minutes or more. Strain and add to a soaking basin.

FULL BODY BATHS: Use the same method as above with larger quantities of herbs. Always prepare the tea separately—bath water isn't hot enough to steep it on its own.

COMPRESSES

Make a double-strength infusion (twice the herbs). Apply warm or refrigerate for a cooling effect. Soak a thin towel or handkerchief in tea and apply it to the affected area. Refrigerated tea keeps for several days and can be reheated.

POULTICES

Place a thin towel in a bowl and add 1 cup of herbs in the center. Add hot water, 1 to 2 tablespoons at a time, until the herbs are warm and moist but not soaking. Gather the towel edges to create an herb bundle. Wring it slightly and apply it to the skin for 10 to 15 minutes. Reuse by drying and rehydrating the herbs.

DOSAGES

Tea

For medicinal dosing of tea, drink about 3 to 4 cups per day (about one pot or a full French press). To brew, for each cup of hot water, mix 1 tablespoon of herb per cup of hot water. Start small when testing blends—mix 1 tablespoon of each herb to create a sample batch.

Tincture

Standard dose: 2 dropperfuls, 2 to 3 times daily. 1 dropperful is approximately 30 drops, so if you buy a bottle that says the dosage is 30 to 90 drops, that means 1 to 3 dropperfuls. To get a dropperful, squeeze the dropper inside the bottle, then release, getting the dropper as full as you can.

Some remedies are used as needed, which usually refers to taking 1 to 2 dropperfuls when you need it (unless otherwise noted).

For sensitive individuals, or when experiencing adverse effects, start with just a few drops and increase the dose gradually. Body chemistry fluctuates—what doesn't work today might work tomorrow.

Oils & Salves

Apply daily as desired. If you're concerned about an allergy, first do a patch test by placing a small amount of the oil or salve on your skin. Wait at least 30 minutes to see if you have any type of negative reaction. If irritation occurs, stop applying the oil or salve and talk to your doctor about potential allergies.

Baths, Soaks & Compresses

Use multiple times daily if desired. Discontinue if your skin becomes irritated or dry.

Poultices

Apply 3 times weekly, or daily if your skin tolerates them well.

LABELING & STORAGE

Labels are essential! For home remedies, I use masking tape to write a label, but you have other options. Write on paper and tape it to jars, or create a remedy notebook with corresponding numbers on containers.

Be sure to include this information on every label:

- Date (month, day, year—I've found mystery jars in my cupboard with no date!)
- Herb name (common and Latin if possible—after years of medicine making, species differences in efficacy and flavor become important)
- Amount used ("1 cup calendula, *Calendula officinalis*" or "1 oz" or "filled jar ⅓ full")
- Menstruum details ("1.5 cups Tito's 80 proof vodka")—if using Everclear and water, note proportions

STORAGE

Teas will keep in the refrigerator for about 3 days before spoiling. Keep them lidded to preserve essential oils.

Store most herbal remedies out of the heat and the sunlight. Light and heat evaporate alcohol from tinctures and degrade other preparations. While some oil recipes suggest sunny windowsills for gentle heating, watch for water condensation that causes mold and rancidity.

Storage Times

TINCTURES & LINIMENTS: Several years in a cool, dark place. Check for plastic dropper erosion or rust on metal lids.

OILS: Up to 2 years in a cool, dark place. Check for mold or rancid smell.

SYRUPS: Refrigerate. With a 1:1 sugar ratio, syrups last 3 months. Reduced-sugar versions with brandy last 1 to 2 months. Check by smelling and by watching for mold.

POULTICE HERBS & COMPRESS TEAS: Compost after use (both can be reused a couple times before disposal).

SAFETY & ETHICS

Seek out community resources to deepen your herbal knowledge! Look for herb walks, nature walks, ethnobotany courses, or classes at local herb shops and natural food stores. Seeing plants in their natural habitat and learning your local flora is invaluable. Always work with experienced foragers before harvesting—they'll teach proper identification and sustainable harvesting practices that allow plants to regenerate.

As herbalists, we must consider sustainability. How can we practice herbal medicine without overusing endangered plants? Check United Plant Savers for information on at-risk species.

OTHER RESOURCES

In Washington state, I recommend Natalie Hammerquist of the Adiantum School of Plant Medicine and Suzanne Tabert of the Cedar Mountain Herb School for outdoor plant learning. The American Herbalist Guild, our national association, offers classes and Registered Herbalist certification.

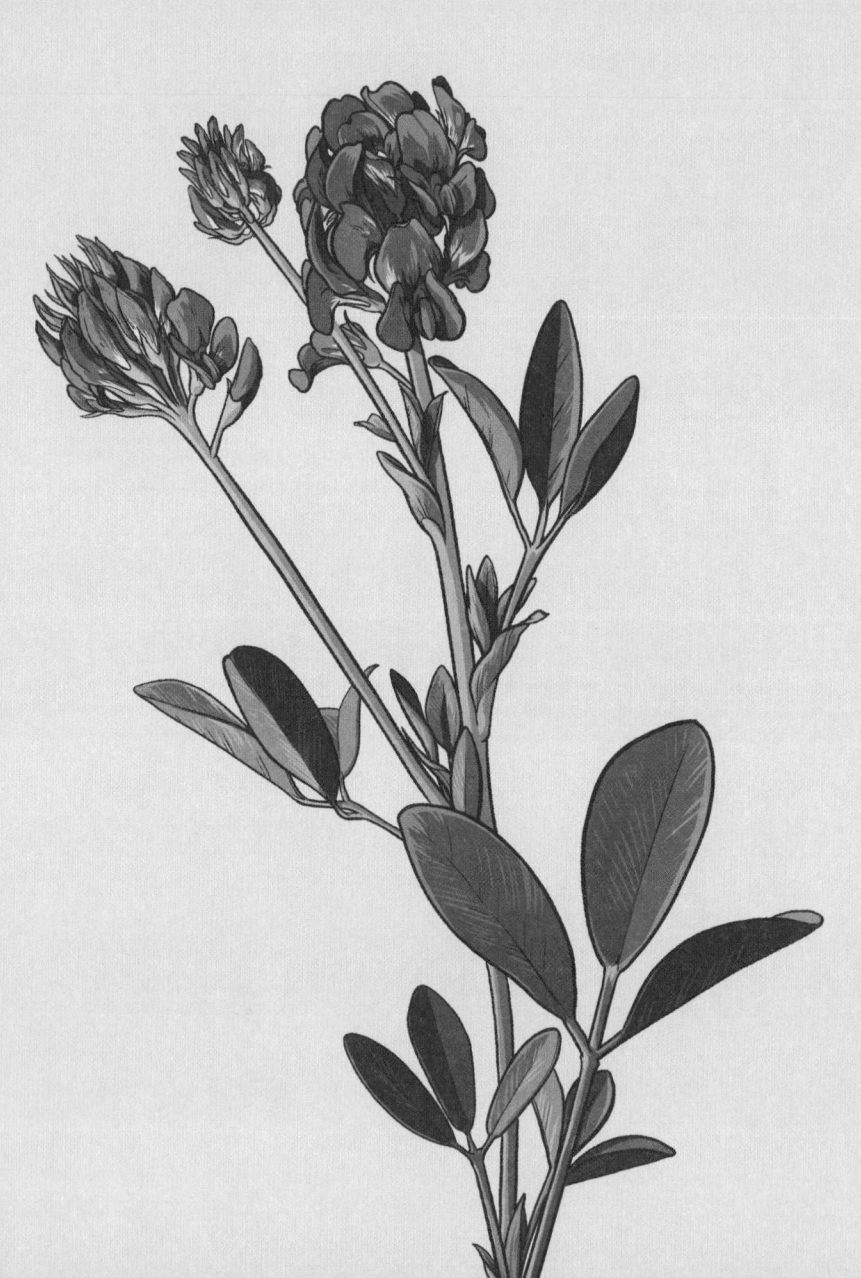

PART 2

100 Remedies for Everyday Ailments

This section contains 100 remedies for everyday ailments and is designed to be multifunctional and educational. Although they are organized alphabetically for easy reference, I encourage you to browse through all the remedies to understand how they can address multiple concerns. As a clinical herbalist, I aim to help people address root causes, not just symptoms. For example, if you catch a cold whenever you're feeling stressed, you can use the stress and anxiety remedies between illnesses for prevention and then use the acute remedies when needed.

Some sections reference other remedies—I'll explain these connections. I'll also note good herb substitutions or what can be omitted while maintaining effectiveness. Most recipes use dried herbs and should be easy to source. If using fresh herbs instead, you'll need larger amounts—see the Making Herbal Medicine section for details.

A few herbs appear in recipes but not in the main herb list. All herbs are medicinal, and there are simply too many to include comprehensively! When a new herb appears in the ailments section, I provide a brief description on first mention.

Acid Reflux

The herbs in this formula help to soothe and cool irritated tissues. While avoiding trigger foods helps, this tea also works as a daily tonic for stomach health.

DOSAGE: 1 to 3 cups of tea per day

INGREDIENTS

1 part marshmallow root

1 part marshmallow leaf

½ part plantain

½ part chamomile

¼ part calendula

¼ part fennel

INSTRUCTIONS: Combine all ingredients and steep for 10 to 15 minutes, using 1 tablespoon of the herb mixture per cup of hot water. Strain and serve.

HOW TO USE: Drink as a daily tonic to soothe irritated stomach tissues.

TIP: If this remedy doesn't relieve reflux symptoms, try the Cold Infused Marshmallow Root for Acid Reflux instead.

REMEDY: COLD INFUSED MARSHMALLOW ROOT FOR ACID REFLUX

Drink daily as a cooling tonic, or sip slowly during symptoms. Marshmallow root, when made as a cold infusion, draws out the mucilaginous components that are gooey and sticky. This texture provides a soothing coating to the esophagus and stomach to cool the burning and help heal the tissues.

DOSAGE: 1 quart daily

INGREDIENTS

4 tablespoons dried marshmallow root

INSTRUCTIONS: Follow the instructions for cold infusions on page 7.

HOW TO USE: After straining the herbs, pour the infusion back into the cleaned jar and drink from it throughout the day.

TIP: Refrigerate unused portions for up to 3 days. Just check for rancidity; it will smell off. You can drink this tea long-term to help repair the lining in your esophagus and stomach.

Acne

Supporting liver detoxification often improves acne significantly. Start here for gentle, effective treatment.

DOSAGE: Drink 1 to 3 cups daily. If skin worsens or stomach upset occurs, reduce the dosage, dilute the tea, or only drink it a few times a week.

INGREDIENTS

1 part red clover buds

1 part spearmint

1 part burdock

1 part dandelion root

1 part plantain

1 part calendula

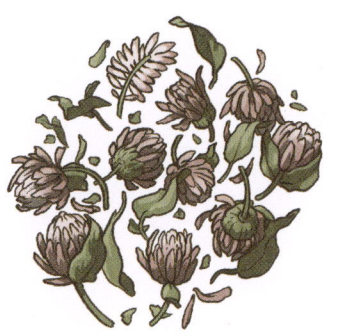

INSTRUCTIONS: Combine all ingredients and steep for 10 to 15 minutes, using 1 tablespoon of the herb mixture per cup of hot water (or less if it's too bitter). Strain and serve.

HOW TO USE: Make it as a tea and sip it warm.

TIP: Add honey for flavor if you'd like. If you're avoiding sugar (or if you notice your skin is reacting to sugar), you can add a pinch of dried stevia leaf to the formula or increase the amount of spearmint. Dried stevia is nutritious and delicious and nothing like the processed substitutes many are familiar with. During breakouts, avoid caffeine, alcohol, fried food, spicy food, and sugar until new lesions stop forming. Once clear, gradually reduce or stop the herbs.

REMEDY: ACNE HEALING VINEGAR

Apple cider vinegar's healing properties intensify with added herbs.

DOSAGE: Use as needed for acne outbreaks.

INGREDIENTS

1.5 cups apple cider vinegar

4 tablespoons rose petals (or buds)

4 tablespoons calendula

2 tablespoons chamomile

3 tablespoons lemon balm

3 tablespoons rosemary

1 tablespoon lavender (optional)

INSTRUCTIONS: Combine all ingredients in a pint-sized (or larger) jar. Lid, shake gently, and label. Store in a cool, dark place for 3 to 4 weeks. Strain and rebottle in a spray or dropper bottle if desired.

HOW TO USE: Apply a small amount to a cotton ball or pad. Dab on lesions or hold briefly (avoid popping the acne!). The initial sting and smell will fade quickly. Apply regular moisturizer afterward, working around the treated spots.

TIP: Vinegar does not need to be refrigerated, but you can place it in the fridge for a cooling effect on the skin. This vinegar is also ingestible—you may take 1 teaspoon or 1 tablespoon daily if you like. Follow good hygiene basics to avoid reactions: daily showers, weekly sheet/pillowcase washing with mild detergents, and minimal chemical products.

Allergies

If congestion and a stuffy head are your main concerns, this tea can dry up excess mucus effectively.

DOSAGE: 1 to 3 cups a day

INGREDIENTS

1 part yerba santa

1 part tulsi

1 part peppermint

½ part nettles

½ part licorice

½ part rose hips

½ part calendula

½ part elderflower

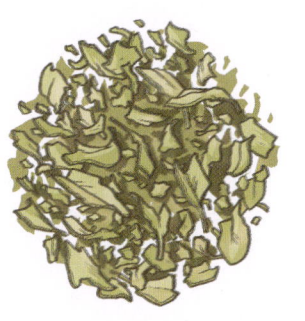

INSTRUCTIONS: Combine all ingredients and steep for 5 to 15 minutes, using 1 tablespoon of the herb mixture per cup of hot water. Strain and serve. Add honey if desired.

HOW TO USE: Make as a tea and drink it warm.

TIP: If there is no congestion, omit the yerba santa. For convenience, convert this recipe into a tincture (buy separate tinctures or follow the tincture recipe in the book to make it yourself), and take 2 dropperfuls up to 3 times a day.

REMEDY: COLD INFUSION NETTLE TEA

Nettles provide natural antihistamine action, which can provide relief for itching, watery eyes, and sneezing.

DOSAGE: 1 quart of tea daily

INGREDIENTS

4 tablespoons nettles

INSTRUCTIONS: Follow instructions for cold infusions on page 7.

HOW TO USE: After straining the herbs back into the infusion jar, you can drink from it throughout the day.

TIP: If you don't finish the tea, refrigerate it for up to 3 days.

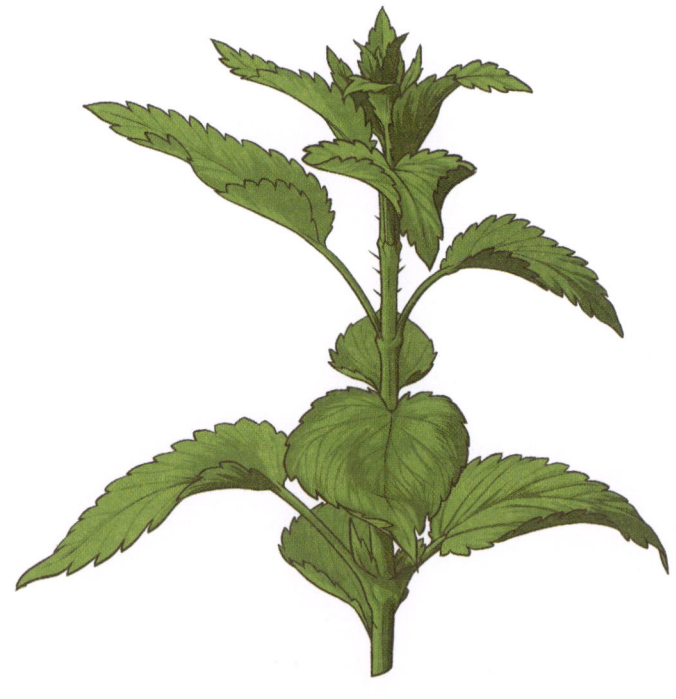

Anal Fissures

REMEDY: SORE BUM SITZ BATH

Sitz baths are excellent home remedies for anal fissures and hemorrhoids, keeping areas clean while simultaneously soothing the tissues. They are often more effective than any topical treatment. Use your bathtub, a low bucket, or (my preference) a toilet sitz bath seat (available online). The latter fits between your toilet seat and bowl.

DOSAGE: Use daily. For severe pain, use up to 3 times a day. Otherwise once daily after your bowel movement is sufficient.

INGREDIENTS

Warm to very warm water

A splash of Epsom salt

INSTRUCTIONS: For the toilet sitz bath, fill the sitz bath seat with warm shower water (hot enough for comfort but not scalding) and add Epsom salt.

For the bathtub, fill the tub 2 to 3 inches deep with warm water and add Epsom salt.

HOW TO USE: Sit in the bath for 10 to 15 minutes. Empty, clean the container, and air or towel dry for next use.

TIP: Plain warm water works well, but calendula baths add healing power. You can steep 4 tablespoons of calendula in 1 quart of hot water for 10 to 15 minutes, strain, add the infusion to your sitz bath, and then soak.

Anemia

This syrup recipe is both effective and pleasant-tasting. While some variations include ingredients such as nutritional yeast or spirulina, this formulation offers a balanced and appealing option without the need for additional components.

DOSAGE: For acute need, use 4 to 6 tablespoons daily. As a general tonic, use 2 to 4 table-spoons daily.

INGREDIENTS

3 tablespoons dandelion root

3 tablespoons dandelion leaf

3 tablespoons nettles

3 tablespoons raspberry leaf

2 tablespoons blackberry leaf

2 tablespoons alfalfa

2 tablespoons yellow dock

1 tablespoon hawthorn berry

2 cups honey

¼ cup brandy

2 tablespoons blackstrap molasses (optional)

INSTRUCTIONS: Follow syrup recipe on page 9.

HOW TO USE: Take directly by mouth. Reduce slightly if the bowels become too loose.

TIP: See the Making Herbal Medicine section for detailed syrup instructions.

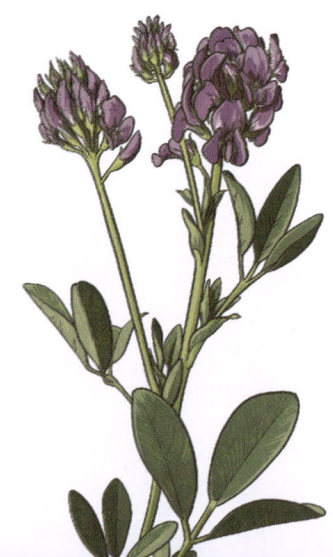

REMEDY: IRON TEA

A pleasant alternative to syrup—use alone or alongside syrup for variety.

DOSAGE: Drink 1 to 3 cups daily. Reduce if your doctor reports you have high iron levels or if your bowels loosen.

INGREDIENTS

1 part blackberry leaf

1 part nettles

1 part raspberry leaf

1 part dandelion root

½ part dandelion leaf

1 part rose hips

INSTRUCTIONS: Combine all ingredients and steep for 10 to 15 minutes, using 1 tablespoon of the herb mixture per cup of hot water. Strain and serve.

HOW TO USE: Make as a tea and drink warm.

TIP: Add honey to taste. For flavor variety, add peppermint, spearmint, or stevia leaf to the dried blend.

REMEDY: YELLOW DOCK TINCTURE

Prepare for bitter medicine! Yellow dock aids digestion, iron assimilation, and hormone health. While not iron-rich like other herbs, it contains above-average iron and supports absorption.

DOSAGE: Take 10 to 30 drops 1 to 3 times per day. Start low to test your tolerance.

INGREDIENTS

Yellow dock dried root

80 to 100 proof vodka (enough to fill your jar)

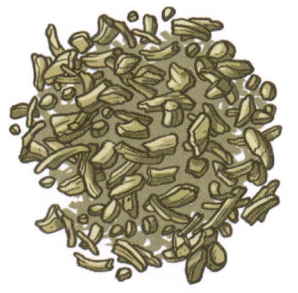

INSTRUCTIONS: Fill a 9-ounce (or up to a pint) jar with a lid halfway with herbs. Cover with alcohol to the top. Label and store in a dry, cool location for 4 weeks, shaking daily. Strain and pour into a clean jar or dropper bottles.

HOW TO USE: Add a dose to a shot glass of water and drink. It is very bitter—chase it with water. Or take it directly by mouth.

TIP: I suggest using smaller jars since yellow dock's bitterness limits its use. At the most, use a pint jar, even if you love it—you can always make more later.

Anxiety

REMEDY: ANXIE-TEA

This tea calms the nervous system beautifully. The ritual itself—prepping herbs, boiling water, watching leaves swirl (the reason I love using a French press)—becomes meditative. Sipping warm liquids soothes your nervous system and energy. In China everyone drank hot water instead of cold— the warmth encourages circulation and slowing down, helping tissues relax rather than constrict.

DOSAGE: Drink 1 cup as needed, up to 4 cups a day.

INGREDIENTS

1 part chamomile

1 part oat straw

1 part lemon verbena

1 part lemon balm

½ part passionflower

INSTRUCTIONS: Combine all ingredients and steep for 10 to 15 minutes, using 1 tablespoon of the herb mixture per cup of hot water. Strain and serve.

HOW TO USE: Make a cup or make a pot. Hold your cup and close your eyes, breathing in the aromatic vapor, and let your mind calm.

TIP: If you don't have oat straw, swap in oat buds. If the tea is too bitter, omit the passionflower.

While drinking the Anxie-Tea as needed or as a daily tonic, keep this tincture handy for faster relief or on-the-go convenience.

DOSAGE: Take a few drops to 2 dropperfuls as needed. Start with a couple of drops, wait 15 minutes to assess the effects, and then increase the dosage if desired.

INGREDIENTS

Passionflower

80 to 100 proof vodka (enough to fill your jar)

INSTRUCTIONS: Fill a jar (up to a pint size) halfway with herbs. Pour in alcohol to the brim and lid, ensuring the herbs stay submerged. Place in a cool, dark place for 4 weeks. Strain.

HOW TO USE: Return the tincture to a cleaned jar and then fill dropper bottles for portability.

TIP: Take in a shot glass with water. Add other calming herbs like chamomile, lavender, or California poppy if desired (maintain same total herb amount).

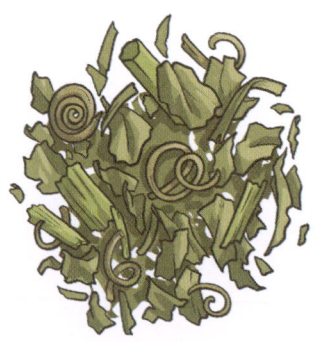

Arthritis

This tea reduces joint pain and inflammation effectively.

DOSAGE: Drink 1 to 3 cups per day as needed.

INGREDIENTS

2 parts nettle

2 parts oat buds or straw

1 part ginger

1 part dandelion root

1 part rosemary

INSTRUCTIONS: Combine all ingredients and steep for 15 minutes, using 1 tablespoon of the herb mixture per cup of hot water. Strain and serve.

HOW TO USE: Drink warm to increase circulation and tissue support.

TIP: Add peppermint, spearmint, stevia, or honey to taste.

Hands are challenging for topical treatments since we use them constantly. This dedicated soak soothes and improves circulation.

DOSAGE: Use daily during discomfort. Reduce frequency if skin becomes irritated.

INGREDIENTS

4 tablespoons of freshly grated ginger

½ gallon of hot water (not scalding)

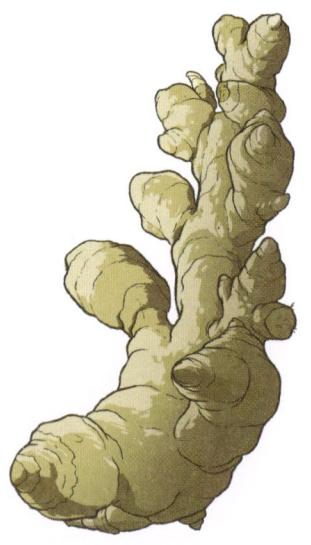

INSTRUCTIONS: Place a large pot or basin near a place where you can sit comfortably. Add grated ginger, and then pour in hot water from the sink or cooled boiled water.

HOW TO USE: Soak your hands until they are pinkish-red. Play with the ginger pieces for a gentle massage. Discard the water after use.

TIP: Avoid if you have open cuts or wounds. For enhanced circulation, try the foot bath from the foot pain section nightly. For a compress alternative, soak a clean towel in ginger tea, wring it out, and apply it to the affected area.

Bloating

This mineral-rich tea with diuretic properties helps with bloating, especially when premenstrual.

DOSAGE: Drink 1 to 2 cups as needed.

INGREDIENTS

1.5 parts dandelion root

1.5 parts dandelion leaf

1 part horsetail

1 part nettle

½ part spearmint

INSTRUCTIONS: Combine all ingredients and steep for 10 to 15 minutes, using 1 tablespoon of the herb mixture per cup of hot water. Strain and serve.

HOW TO USE: Make as a tea and drink it warm.

TIP: If you're feeling bloated due to overeating or digestive discomfort, try the Anxie-Tea or the Tummy Ease Tea instead.

Blood Sugar Stabilization

This tea stabilizes blood sugar and may improve sleep while reducing sweet cravings.

DOSAGE: Drink 1 to 3 cups per day.

INGREDIENTS

1 part cassia chips (cinnamon)

1 part burdock root

1 part marshmallow root

1 part dandelion root

½ part ginger

½ part fenugreek

INSTRUCTIONS: Combine all ingredients and steep for 10 to 15 minutes, using 1 tablespoon of the herb mixture per cup of hot water. Strain and serve.

HOW TO USE: Make as a tea and drink warm.

TIP: Cassia chips (small cinnamon pieces) work best for tea blends—large sticks don't steep well. Roasted dandelion root adds excellent flavor if available.

Bone Strength

This fortifying, mineral-rich tea supports long-term bone and connective tissue health. If you have joint pain, arthritis, or other pain issues, consider taking this in tandem with their alleviating remedies.

DOSAGE: Drink 1 to 3 cups daily.

INGREDIENTS

1 part nettles

1 part oat straw or oat buds

1 part horsetail

1 part gotu kola

1 part peppermint

½ part raspberry leaf

½ part alfalfa

½ part licorice

INSTRUCTIONS: Combine all ingredients and steep for 15 to 30 minutes, using 1 tablespoon of the herb mixture per cup of hot water. Strain and serve.

HOW TO USE: Drink as a hot tea or "steep it and forget it"—let it cool to room temperature.

TIP: If the licorice taste is too strong, omit it or reduce steeping time.

Brain Fog

This is my favorite caffeine-free pick-me-up! Aromatic mints clear your head while gotu kola and ginkgo boost brain circulation.

DOSAGE: Drink 1 cup as needed, up to 3 cups a day.

INGREDIENTS

1 part peppermint

1 part spearmint

1 part gotu kola

1 part gingko

½ part tulsi

INSTRUCTIONS: Combine all ingredients and steep for 5 to 15 minutes, using 1 tablespoon of the herb mixture per cup of hot water. Strain and serve.

HOW TO USE: Make as a tea and drink warm.

TIP: With aromatic blends like this, as the tea is steeping, inhale the vapor and take deep breaths for calm. The healing aromatics enter your sinuses and help wake you up.

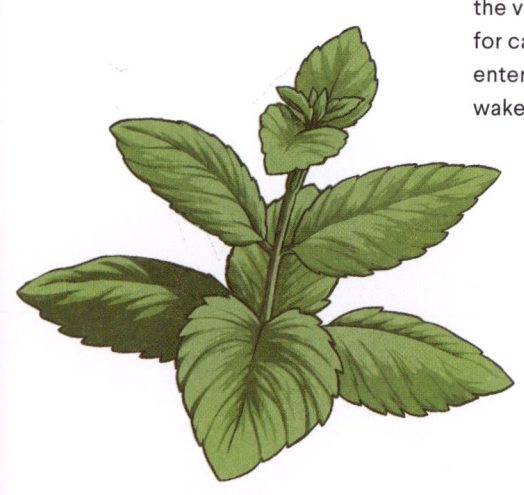

Bug Bites

This folk remedy works wonderfully for mosquito, flea, and no-see-um bites.

DOSAGE: Use as needed for itching, burning, and stinging.

INGREDIENTS

Fresh plantain leaves

Water

Your mouth!

INSTRUCTIONS: Pick plantain leaves (ensure correct identification) from unsprayed areas. Rinse if desired and then chew into a paste.

HOW TO USE: Apply plantain paste directly on the bite, leaving it until dry. It will fall off naturally outdoors, so there is no need to wash it off.

TIP: Baking soda paste also works well. Though I rarely prescribe essential oils, a dab of lavender or peppermint oil can help.

REMEDY: THE BEST BUG SPRAY!

Mosquitoes have loved me since childhood. After trying countless recipes, this is the only one that truly works! I even use it before bed when camping or during summer heat waves in my city apartment.

DOSAGE: Spray generously on your skin, avoiding your eyes. For face application, spray into your palm and pat on.

INGREDIENTS

2 ounces witch hazel

2 ounces water

Equal parts of these essential oils:

Eucalyptus citriodora

Rosemary

Rose geranium

Lavender angustifolia (or lavender spike)

Clove

INSTRUCTIONS: Add 10 drops of each essential oil (only 5 drops of clove initially) to a 4-ounce glass spray bottle. Ensure spray tube reaches bottle bottom. Add witch hazel and water, mix, and spray. Adjust levels as needed.

HOW TO USE: Spray whenever pests threaten. Carry for reapplication outdoors.

TIP: Clove oil irritates skin—never apply it directly. Start with less and then add more if it's tolerated. You can substitute rose water (hydrosol) for water for an amazing scent.

Bruises

Topical applications—especially liniments—are often underutilized in herbal practice. This witch hazel liniment is gentle on the skin and makes a soothing treatment for bruises.

DOSAGE: Apply as frequently as desired after bruising.

INGREDIENTS

1 part mugwort

1 part comfrey

1 part calendula

1 part lavender

Slightly less than 1 pint witch hazel

INSTRUCTIONS: Fill a pint jar (with lid) halfway with dried herbs. Pour in the witch hazel to the top. Lid and shake gently. After 3 to 4 weeks, strain into a clean jar or transfer to dropper/ spray bottles.

HOW TO USE: Place drops in your palm or on a cotton ball. Rub gently on bruises in 3 to 5 layers. Air dry between applications. Reapply several times daily.

TIP: Alcohol can substitute for witch hazel, creating a tincture version. Do not take it internally.

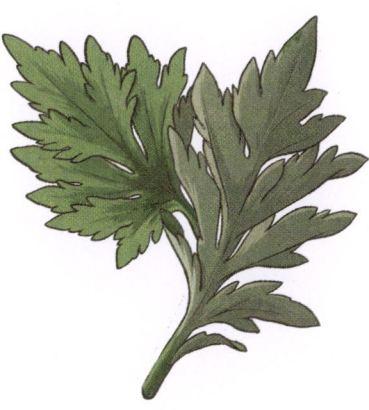

Cholesterol

These herbs help break down fats and improve circulation.

DOSAGE: Drink 1 to 3 cups daily.

INGREDIENTS

2 parts burdock root

2 parts dandelion root

1 part alfalfa

1 part hawthorn berry

1 part hawthorn leaf & flower

1 part ginger

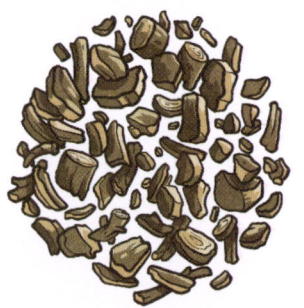

INSTRUCTIONS: Combine all ingredients and steep for 15 to 30 minutes, using 1 tablespoon of the herb mixture per cup of hot water. Strain and serve.

HOW TO USE: Drink daily while managing cholesterol.

TIP: Combine with proper hydration, balanced diet, and exercise for best results. High cholesterol can be genetic—discuss the issue with your doctor.

Circulation

REMEDY: FOOT SOAK FOR BETTER CIRCULATION

I've had cold hands and feet for as long as I remember. In acupuncture school we learned that foot soaks help insomnia by drawing energy (Qi) down from the head. (Have you noticed how cold feet correlate with sleep troubles?) This soak improves circulation wonderfully.

DOSAGE: Soak nightly until circulation improves.

TOOLS

Basin or pot for ankle-deep soaking

Warm to hot water

Towel

INSTRUCTIONS: Fill a basin with warm to hot water (don't scald!). Soak your feet up to your ankles for 10 to 15 minutes until slightly pink. Dry thoroughly. Use thin cotton socks to maintain warmth.

HOW TO USE: See instructions above.

TIP: Adding Epsom salts is optional. You can also steep a single herb—such as rosemary or freshly grated ginger—in a French press to create an herbal tea, similar to the one used in the arthritis soak, and add it to your foot bath. The key therapeutic element is the warm water soak itself; the herbs are a beneficial but nonessential addition.

These herbs improve circulation while warming you thoroughly.

DOSAGE: Drink 1 to 3 cups daily as needed.

INGREDIENTS

2 parts ginger

1 part tulsi

1 part cinnamon

1 part rosemary

1 part hawthorn berry

½ part licorice

INSTRUCTIONS: Combine all ingredients and steep for 10 minutes, using 1 tablespoon of the herb mixture per cup of hot water. Strain and serve.

HOW TO USE: Make as a tea and drink warm.

TIP: A simpler ginger tea can sometimes do the trick! Consider slicing ginger into small discs, and then simmer the ginger in a saucepan with 1 to 2 cups of water for about 20 minutes. Strain and add honey to taste.

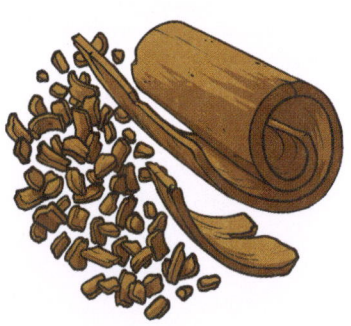

Cold Sores

Herpes is a viral infection, and antiviral herbs can be a supportive part of treatment. This tincture may help prevent an outbreak or shorten its duration.

DOSAGE: Drink 1 to 3 cups a day as needed.

INGREDIENTS

1 part St. John's wort

1 part lemon balm

1 part licorice

1 part calendula

INSTRUCTIONS: Combine all ingredients and steep for 10 to 15 minutes, using 1 tablespoon of the herb mixture per cup of hot water. Strain and serve.

HOW TO USE: Drink this tea if you feel an outbreak approaching.

TIP: If stress tends to trigger your outbreaks, you can also drink the Stress Relief Tea.

Common Cold

Patients have used variations of this effective tea for years!

DOSAGE: Drink 3 to 4 cups daily during symptoms.

INGREDIENTS

1 part peppermint

½ part elderflower

½ part elderberry

¼ part ginger

¼ part cinnamon

¼ part rose hips

INSTRUCTIONS: Combine all ingredients and steep for 15 to 30 minutes, using 1 tablespoon of the herb mixture per cup of hot water. Strain and serve.

HOW TO USE: Drink warm to hot. Add honey if desired.

TIP: Make a pot and drink over several hours while sick. For early symptoms (fever, stiff neck), see the Fever section on page 67. For coughing or congestion, refer to those sections—alternate or combine remedies.

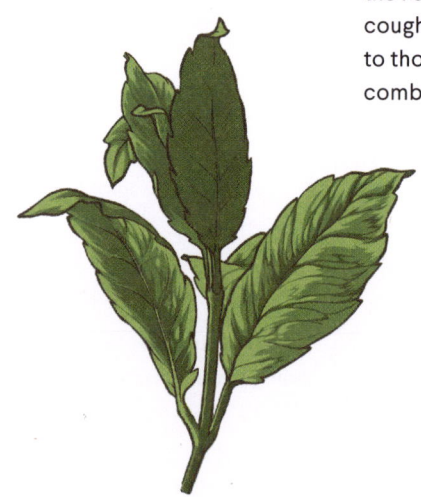

REMEDY: COLD KICKING VINEGAR

Sometimes called "Fire Cider," this medicinal vinegar with vegetables and herbs boosts immunity at the first signs of a cold. It also helps thin and expectorate phlegm. Try as daily immune tonic on salads.

DOSAGE: Take 1 tablespoon 3 to 4 times daily at the first sign of cold.

INGREDIENTS

1 quart of apple cider vinegar

1 onion

1 head of garlic

1 large knob of ginger (peeled, chopped/grated)

¼ to ⅓ cup horseradish (peeled, chopped/grated)

1 lemon (quartered, squeezed)

1 pinch of cayenne

2 sprigs of fresh rosemary (or 1 tablespoon dried)

2 sprigs of fresh thyme (or 1 tablespoon dried)

Honey

INSTRUCTIONS: Chop the vegetables. Layer them in a 1-quart jar, pressing down, until the jar is three-fourths full. Add herbs and lemon. Fill three-fourths full with vinegar. You can also add honey to the remaining space, but this is optional. (If you opt out of the honey, then fill the jar all the way to the top with vinegar instead.) Press down with a spoon. Lid, label, and store in a cool dark place for 3 to 4 weeks. Strain. You can eat the vegetables like pickles!

HOW TO USE: Take vinegar straight or diluted. Store pickled vegetables in the refrigerator. The vinegar needs no refrigeration.

OPTIONAL ADDITIONS: 1 chopped jalapeno (destemmed and mostly deseeded), fresh or dried sage, fresh turmeric, dried astragalus, dried hibiscus, dried hawthorn berries, fresh orange

TIP: Experiment! I love adding orange, hibiscus (high in vitamin C, astringent, and immune-supporting), and astragalus to the base.

Congestion

Herbal steams are wonderfully soothing and effective for congestion relief.

DOSAGE: Add 2 to 3 heaping tablespoons of dried herbs to about 2 cups of hot water (the exact water amount isn't critical, just ensure the bowl isn't full so you can position your face above it).

INGREDIENTS

Use equal parts of any or all

1 part eucalyptus

1 part rosemary

1 part peppermint

1 part thyme

1 part sage

1 part yarrow

INSTRUCTIONS: Start by mixing 1 tablespoon of each herb in a small jar to test the blend and see how you like it. When you're ready to steam, place 3 to 4 tablespoons of herb in a bowl near a comfortable seating area. Next pour 1 to 2 cups of boiling water over the herbs.

HOW TO USE: Sit with your head over the bowl and a towel draped around your head. Set a timer for 5 to 10 minutes. Breathe the vapor through your nose. If it's too hot, wait briefly, but try to capture those aromatic oils while they're warm.

TIP: Let the water cool before straining it into the sink. Discard the herbs in the compost. This steam also relaxes the nervous system when you feel ill. Use whatever herbs you have available!

Constipation

REMEDY: EASY MOVER TEA

For occasional sluggish bowels, this tea gently relaxes the tummy and bowels without forcing movement. Unlike teas containing senna or cascara bark (which cause colon contractions and can be harmful long term), this blend works mildly.

DOSAGE: Drink 1 to 2 cups in the evening before bed. Daytime use is fine since urgency is uncommon.

INGREDIENTS

2 parts chamomile

1 part marshmallow root

1 part ginger

½ part fennel

½ part licorice

INSTRUCTIONS: Combine all ingredients and steep for 10 to 15 minutes, using 1 tablespoon of the herb mixture per cup of hot water. Strain and serve.

HOW TO USE: Drink before bed to relax the nervous system and promote easier morning movements.

TIP: This remedy may take several days to yield results.

OTHER REMEDIES: Try the Herbal Iron Syrup and the Yellow Dock Tincture from the Anemia section or the Castor Oil Pack remedy from the Liver section.

Cough

REMEDY: COUGH SYRUP

This syrup works for any cough type, but it's particularly helpful for wet coughs.

DOSAGE: Take 1 to 2 teaspoons every hour throughout the day or as needed. Continue taking even after improvement.

INGREDIENTS

4 parts fennel

2 parts licorice

2 parts marshmallow root

2 parts mullein

2 parts elecampane

1 part cinnamon

½ part ginger

¼ part orange peel

1 to 2 cups of cane sugar or honey

¼ cup brandy (optional)

INSTRUCTIONS: Follow syrup recipe on page 9.

HOW TO USE: Take the dosage straight in the mouth; for a sore throat, let it linger momentarily.

TIP: For a spasmodic cough, add 1 part valerian root. Orange peel adds vitamin C, astringency, and a pleasant flavor.

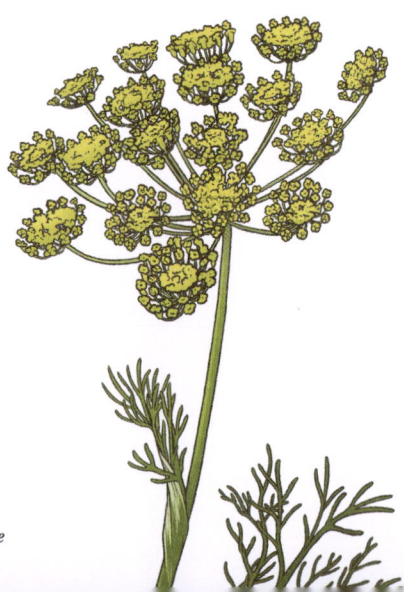

REMEDY: DRY COUGH TEA

Whether your coughs start dry or linger, this soothes mucous membranes and nourishes lung tissue.

DOSAGE: Drink up to 3 cups daily while symptoms persist.

INGREDIENTS

1 part mullein

1 part marshmallow root

1 part marshmallow leaf

½ part peppermint

¼ part licorice

¼ part cinnamon

¼ part fennel

INSTRUCTIONS: Combine all ingredients and steep for 15 to 30 minutes, using 1 tablespoon of the herb mixture per cup of hot water. Strain and serve. Add honey to taste.

HOW TO USE: Continue drinking daily for at least 2 weeks, as dry coughs heal slowly.

TIP: Add 1 part elecampane if phlegm persists, or take the cough syrup above in smaller doses (2 to 3 times daily instead of every hour).

REMEDY: PEAR COMPOTE FOR DRY LUNGS

Chinese medicine food therapy proves invaluable during recovery. Pears nourish lung yin tissue beautifully (apples work too).

DOSAGE: About 1 pear daily

INGREDIENTS

1 to 2 pears (any variety)

Freshly squeezed lemon juice (from about half of a lemon)

Splash of maple syrup

Optional: rosemary or thyme

INSTRUCTIONS: Chop pears into 1-inch cubes (leave skin on). Heat in a saucepan on medium, adding just enough water to prevent burning. Simmer without boiling. Stir frequently. As the pears soften, add lemon juice and a splash of maple syrup to taste. Simmer for 15 minutes until mushy. Mash to desired consistency.

HOW TO USE: Eat from the bowl, or add it to oatmeal or yogurt.

TIP: The compote can be refrigerated for 2 to 3 days.

Cramps

Whether you're about to get your period or you're on your menstrual cycle, this formula eases menstrual discomfort.

DOSAGE: Drink 1 cup as needed for menstrual cramps.

INGREDIENTS

1 part cramp bark

1 part chamomile

1 part raspberry leaf

½ part ginger

½ part rose petals

INSTRUCTIONS: Combine all ingredients and steep for 10 minutes, using 1 tablespoon of the herb mixture per cup of hot water. Strain and serve.

HOW TO USE: Make as a tea and drink warm.

TIP: If bitter, the rose petals may be the culprit. Steep for less time or add the roses after the initial steeping for a shorter extraction.

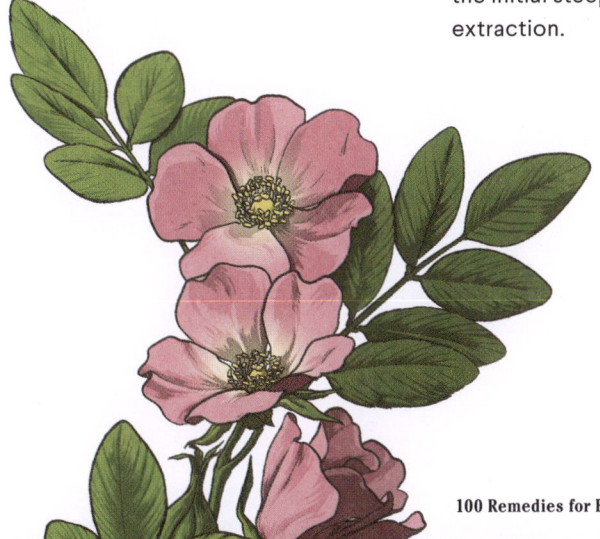

REMEDY: CRAMP EASE ELIXIR

How often have cramps struck when you're away from home—in the car, at work, at the gym? This portable tincture provides reliable relief.

DOSAGE: Take 1 to 2 dropperfuls every 15 to 30 minutes as needed.

INGREDIENTS

1 part cramp bark

1 part chamomile

1 part black cohosh

2 cups of brandy

¼ cup of honey

INSTRUCTIONS: Fill a pint jar halfway with the herbs. Add brandy to the jar until it's three-fourths full and add honey to fill. Lid, and then shake gently or stir (honey requires persistent stirring). Label and steep for 3 to 4 weeks in a cool, dark place.

HOW TO USE: Take directly by mouth. When traveling without mixing supplies, hold some water in your mouth, add tincture, and swallow.

TIP: Add a little bit of rose to this formula for additional support.

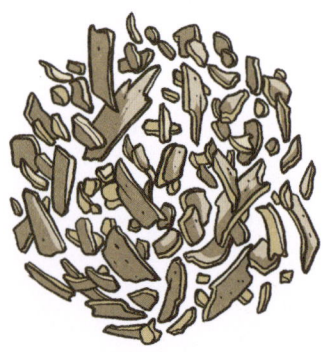

Dehydration

Sometimes plain water doesn't hydrate enough in hot weather or post workout. This mineral-rich tea beats sugary electrolyte drinks.

DOSAGE: Drink 1 quart daily or as desired.

INGREDIENTS

2 tablespoons marshmallow root

2 tablespoons spearmint

INSTRUCTIONS: Add herbs to a 1-quart jar and fill with room temperature water. Lid and refrigerate for 4 hours to overnight. Strain (slight mucilage is beneficial) and drink.

HOW TO USE: Drink like water throughout the day!

TIP: If the mucilaginous texture bothers you, reduce steeping time or substitute marshmallow leaf. Alternatively make a hot infusion. Adding 1 teaspoon to 1 tablespoon of chia seeds (even to plain water) provides extra hydration (they'll float rather than thicken).

Depression

For those days when you're feeling down, or for bouts of depression (sadness, loss of joy in usual activities, or fatigue), try these uplifting herbs. Damiana, often labeled an aphrodisiac, works as a mild antidepressant. Oat straw and lemon balm calm and nourish nerves. Rose moves stagnant Qi—that stuck feeling. Effects may be immediate or require regular use.

DOSAGE: Drink 1 to 3 cups daily as needed.

INGREDIENTS

2 parts oat straw

1 part damiana

1 part gingko

½ part lemon balm

½ part rose

INSTRUCTIONS: Combine all ingredients and steep for 10 minutes, using 1 tablespoon of the herb mixture per cup of hot water. Strain and serve.

HOW TO USE: Make as a tea and drink warm.

TIP: For serious depression, consult your healthcare provider. As a clinician I encourage all physically able patients to walk 30 minutes daily (minimum 3 times weekly). Movement, fresh air, nature observation, and exercise benefit brain chemistry over time. Try walking without your headphones—let your mind clear and notice nature.

REMEDY: ST. JOHN'S WORT TINCTURE

St. John's wort provides gentle antidepressant action. Its flowers bloom around June in sunny fields. Hold the leaves to the light to see tiny holes letting sunshine through—reflecting how it makes you feel!

DOSAGE: Take 1 dropperful 3 times daily. Adjust for any sensitivity—a few drops may suffice.

INGREDIENTS

Freshly harvested St. John's wort flower tops (a few stems and leaves are okay)

1.5 to 2 cups of 80 to 100 proof vodka (enough to cover)

INSTRUCTIONS: Harvest the flowers through classes, farms, or community connections. The ideal harvest timing is when partially closed blooms release a red liquid when squeezed. Wilt the flowers overnight on a table. Fill a pint jar three-fourths full with the flowers and cover with the alcohol. Label and store for 4 weeks in a cool, dry place. Shake regularly.

HOW TO USE: Take directly in your mouth, or use the shot glass method.

TIP: Fresh St. John's wort isn't convenient, but dried flowers lack effectiveness. It may take up to 1 month to experience full effects.

Diarrhea

Diarrhea can be caused by bacterial or viral infections or by spoiled food. Blackberry root tincture can be difficult to find, but you can make your own. Neighbors may appreciate your help taming their blackberry patches.

DOSAGE: Take 1 to 2 dropperfuls 2 to 4 times daily as needed.

INGREDIENTS

Blackberry root bark (fresh or dried)

Alcohol (80 to 100 proof vodka)

INSTRUCTIONS: Harvest carefully with gloves, digging out the roots with tools. Clean roots and peel the bark with a sharp knife (vegetable peelers won't work). Chop the bark and fill an 8-ounce jar halfway. Cover with alcohol. Lid, shake, and label. Steep for 3 to 4 weeks in a cool, dark place. Strain into dropper bottles.

HOW TO USE: Take directly in your mouth or with a little shot of water.

TIP: See your doctor if symptoms worsen, fever persists, blood appears in your stool, or you're concerned. Resulting dehydration can be serious.

REMEDY: REHYDRATING TEA FOR THE RUNS

Augment the tincture with this hydrating tea. If you lack dried blackberry root, use the leaf instead.

DOSAGE: Consume a 1-quart pot through the day.

INGREDIENTS

2 parts blackberry leaf or root

1 part spearmint

1 part marshmallow leaf

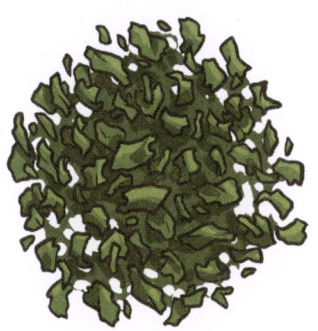

INSTRUCTIONS: Combine all ingredients and steep for 15 to 30 minutes (less time if it gets too astringent or bitter), using ¼ cup of dried herb per quart of hot water. Strain and serve.

HOW TO USE: Sip throughout the day to avoid dehydration.

TIP: See your doctor if symptoms worsen, fever persists, blood appears in your stool, or you're concerned. Resulting dehydration can be serious.

Digestion

This tea soothes sensitive stomachs, bloating, overeating, or stomach cramps effectively.

DOSAGE: Drink 1 cup as needed, up to 3 cups daily.

INGREDIENTS

1 part chamomile

1 part peppermint

1 part oat buds

½ part licorice

½ part fennel

½ part ginger

INSTRUCTIONS: Combine all ingredients and steep for 10 minutes, using 1 tablespoon of the herb mixture per cup of hot water. Strain and serve.

HOW TO USE: Make as a tea and drink warm.

TIP: As with any of these tea blends, try individual herbs on their own to understand their unique tastes and effects—this helps when modifying formulas.

REMEDY: SOOTHING TUMMY GUMMIES

Homemade gummies provide gut-soothing benefits! Gelatin reduces gut inflammation, while chamomile and rose add anti-inflammatory, soothing properties.

DOSAGE: Start with consuming 2 to 3 gummies to assess tolerance. One pan of gummies can last several days.

INGREDIENTS

3 heaping tablespoons of chamomile

1 heaping tablespoon of rose

4 tablespoons of grass-fed gelatin

2 tablespoons honey

A small amount of coconut oil

INSTRUCTIONS: Steep 4 tablespoons of the herbs in 2 cups water for 15 minutes (it should be strong but not bitter). Meanwhile, add gelatin to 2.5 ounces of room temperature water to bloom. Strain the tea into the gelatin mixture and whisk gently. Add honey. Grease a shallow glass pan (8x8 is preferable) lightly with coconut oil. Pour the mixture into the pan and refrigerate for 2 hours or until firm. Cut into 2 x 2 squares, and then store in an airtight container in the refrigerator.

HOW TO USE: Eat alone as a treat!

TIP: You can try other combinations such as elderberry-ginger for immunity or nettle for a pale-green color. Use 2 tablespoons of gelatin for a softer texture. Introduce gradually to avoid constipation.

Dreaming

For interesting dream experiences, sip this before bed. Mugwort traditionally aids in dream recall, but it can also enhance your dreams! Its effects vary by person.

DOSAGE: Take 1 to 2 tablespoons 1 hour before bed.

INGREDIENTS

½ cup mugwort

2 heaping tablespoons of damiana

1 cinnamon stick or 1 teaspoon of cassia chips

1 cup of brandy

¼ to ½ cup honey

INSTRUCTIONS: Combine herbs and brandy in jar with ¼ cup of honey. Lid and shake. Steep for 2 weeks in a cool, dry place. Taste and add remaining honey if desired. Steep for 1 more week. Strain into a clean jar.

HOW TO USE: Sip from a small cordial glass while winding down at the end of the day.

TIP: Keep a dream journal next to your bed so that you can record dreams upon waking. This practice helps you remember.

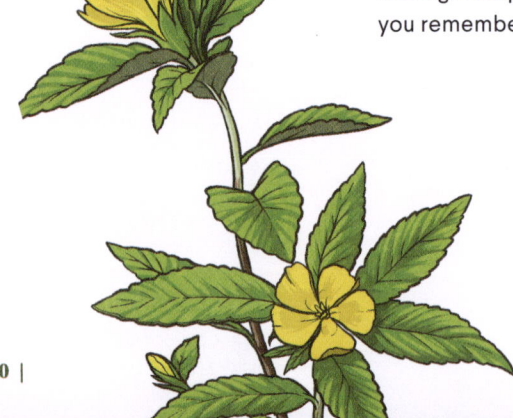

Dry Skin

These cooling, moisturizing herbs soothe itchy, irritated skin. Remember that excessive bathing dries the skin—maintain hydration and topical moisture.

DOSAGE: Take 1 bath as needed (not daily as it may overdry your skin). Combine with hydration and topical moisturizing.

INGREDIENTS

1 part chamomile

1 part calendula

1 part marshmallow root

1 part fennel

1 part rose (totaling ½ cup)

INSTRUCTIONS: Herbs should total about 1.5 cups. Add herbs to a ½-gallon jar and pour boiling water over them to fill. Cover to retain the oils. Steep for 10 to 15 minutes while filling your tub. Strain directly into your bath and hop in while it's warm.

HOW TO USE: Soak in the warm herbal bath, feeling the moisturizing effects.

TIP: Apply the Herbal Skin Oil for Dry Skin to your skin directly after the bath to enhance the benefits!

REMEDY: HERBAL SKIN OIL FOR DRY SKIN

Moisturizing your body with oil can make for a lovely ritual. Apply after bathing while your skin is slightly damp, as the water and oil together help absorption.

DOSAGE: Apply as desired.

INGREDIENTS

1 cup of herbs (1 part calendula, 1 part lavender, and 1 part chamomile)

1 cup of grapeseed or olive oil

1 to 2 teaspoons of vodka

INSTRUCTIONS: Using a 1-quart jar and a muslin cloth for straining, follow the alcohol-intermediary method for making herbal oils on page 10.

HOW TO USE: After bathing, start with a dime-sized amount—a little goes a long way! Massage from arms to feet, focusing on stiff or dry areas. Wear old pajamas if you're concerned about staining.

TIP: See page 9 for other methods of making herbal oils.

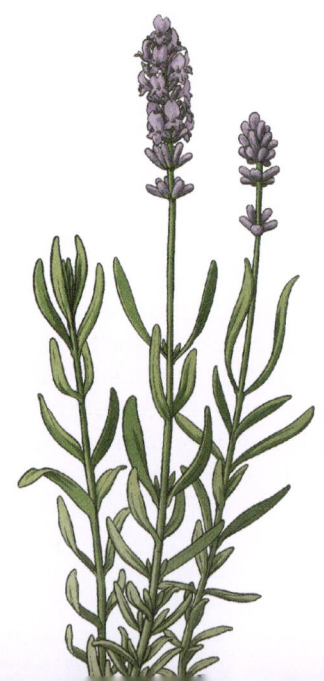

Earache

Infections of the ear can be bacterial or viral—I refer patients to doctors, especially if blood appears on the pillow. Try these remedies in the early stages, while drinking Fever Diminish Tea simultaneously if you have a fever. This oil relieves pain and helps fight infection.

DOSAGE: Take 3 to 4 drops 3 times daily.

INGREDIENTS

2 to 3 tablespoons of chopped fresh garlic

2 to 3 tablespoons of dried mullein flowers

Olive oil

INSTRUCTIONS: Make this fresh on the stove. Combine garlic and mullein in a double boiler with just enough oil to cover. Warm for 30 minutes without boiling. Strain through cheesecloth-lined mesh into a measuring cup. Squeeze out the oil and transfer to a dropper bottle. Warm slightly in your hands or float the bottle in hot water before use (avoid water entering the bottle).

HOW TO USE: Place 3 to 4 drops directly into your ear. Massage around the ear gently (front, back, and around). Lie down briefly. Keep a cotton pad nearby for drips. Refrigerate between uses.

TIP: Mullein flowers are harvested in the spring and fall. Ask at local herb shops or farms about their availability. For additional relief, wrap a heating pad in a small towel and rest your ear on it on a pillow. This remedy is often available at natural food stores if you're unable to make it.

Eczema

Skin conditions often benefit from liver support, but identifying your individual triggers is crucial. Address your underlying triggers by referring to relevant sections in this book.

DOSAGE: Drink 3 cups daily as needed.

INGREDIENTS

1 part burdock

1 part calendula

1 part red clover

1 part nettles

INSTRUCTIONS: Combine all ingredients and steep for 10 to 15 minutes, using 1 tablespoon of the herb mixture per cup of hot water. Strain and serve.

HOW TO USE: Make as a tea and drink warm.

TIP: Try compresses of burdock, witch hazel, or calendula for topical relief.

Eye Strain

This compress relieves minor eye strain with cooling, soothing effects.

DOSAGE: Apply 1 to 2 times daily.

INGREDIENTS

2 tablespoons calendula flowers

INSTRUCTIONS: Use 2 tablespoons of flowers per cup of hot water. Steep for 15 to 20 minutes and then strain. Cool to slightly warm or refrigerate for a cold compress.

HOW TO USE: Soak a thin, clean tea towel in the liquid, wring it out, and place it over your eyes while reclining. Alternatively lean over the sink, scoop the liquid into a clean palm, and cup it over your eye briefly.

TIP: Always ensure your hands are clean before performing any eye treatments.

Fatigue

Lemon verbena's calming yet tart nature provides gentle energy. These combined herbs improve focus and circulation—a nutritive pick-me-up!

DOSAGE: Drink 1 cup as needed.

INGREDIENTS

1 part lemon verbena

1 part gotu kola

1 part ginkgo

1 part hawthorn berry

½ part orange peel

INSTRUCTIONS: Combine all ingredients and steep for 15 minutes, using 1 heaping tablespoon of the herb mixture per cup of hot water. Strain and serve.

HOW TO USE: Make as a tea and serve warm.

TIP: Adjust herbs based on what's available.

Fever

Fevers can be scary, but they help your body fight illness. Contact your doctor if your fever persists without improvement. When you're feeling poorly, sipping this throughout the day will work better than forcing down large amounts.

DOSAGE: Drink 1 to 4 cups of tea daily.

INGREDIENTS

1 part yarrow

1 part peppermint

1 part elderflowers

INSTRUCTIONS: Combine all ingredients and steep for 15 minutes, using 1 tablespoon of the herb mixture per cup of hot water. Strain and serve.

HOW TO USE: Make as a tea and drink warm.

TIP: Combine with symptom-specific remedies from other sections.

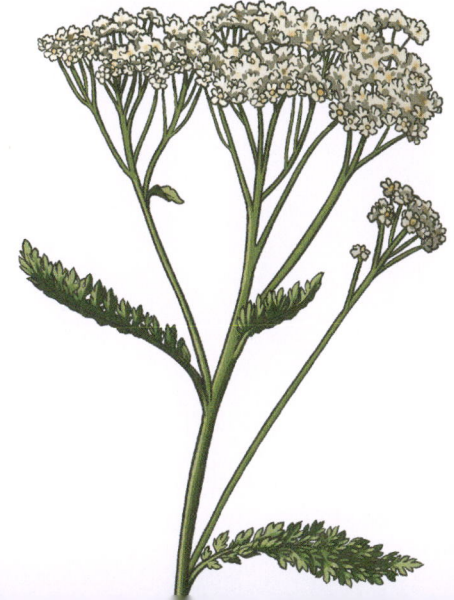

Foot Pain

This foot soak soothes sore, tired feet beautifully. Try peppermint, chamomile, lemon balm, or rosemary variations. For plantar fasciitis, regular soaks and massage provide surprising relief.

DOSAGE: Soak daily if desired.

INGREDIENTS

1 part calendula

1 part comfrey

1 part lavender

A few tablespoons of Epsom salt (optional)

INSTRUCTIONS: Make a strong tea, using ¼ cup of herbs to 1 quart of water. Steep for 15 minutes or more, and then strain into a foot basin. Add more warm water (and Epsom salt if using). Make sure it's a comfortable temperature—don't scald your feet. Soak for 15 to 20 minutes until your feet turn pink.

HOW TO USE: Often this is best at the end of the day for ultimate relaxation, though you can soak any time.

TIP: Follow with an herbal oil foot massage, put on socks, and head to bed. This is a lovely bedtime ritual!

Gas

REMEDY: GOODBYE GAS TEA

Carminative herbs help reduce or prevent gas—you probably know these herbs but may not realize this is a primary function.

DOSAGE: Drink 1 cup as needed.

INGREDIENTS

1 part chamomile

1 part fennel

1 part ginger

1 part peppermint

(Choose 1 herb or mix equal parts of your preferred herbs)

INSTRUCTIONS: Combine all ingredients and steep for 10 minutes, using 1 tablespoon of the herb mixture per cup of hot water. Strain and serve.

HOW TO USE: Make as a tea and drink warm.

TIP: Regular use prevents gas. Hot tea provides the best relief during acute discomfort.

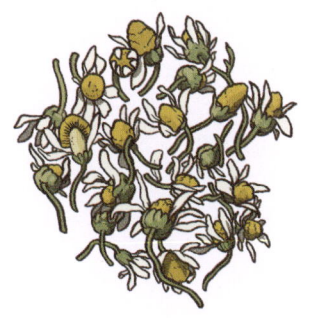

General Health Tonics

This nutritive tea serves as my daily multivitamin—I swap herbs based on mood and needs!

DOSAGE: Drink 1 to 4 cups a day as needed for an extra boost of vitamins and minerals.

INGREDIENTS

1 part nettles

1 part rose hips

1 part oat straw

½ part peppermint

½ part dandelion root or leaf

½ part red clover blossoms

INSTRUCTIONS: Combine all ingredients and steep for 15 to 30 minutes, using 1 tablespoon of the herb mixture per cup of hot water. Strain and serve.

HOW TO USE: Make as a tea and drink warm, or let it cool down and sip throughout the day as a water replacement.

TIP: I often steep this while getting ready for the day. Then I pour it into a large to-go container for all-day sipping. You can also make it the night before and refrigerate.

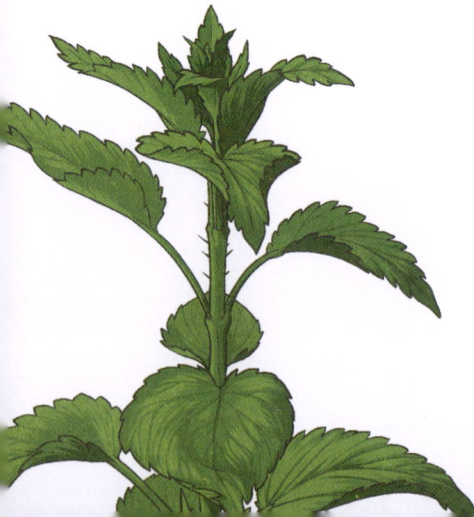

REMEDY: ROOT BEER SYRUP

Inspired by a childhood love of root beer, this herbal version offers a naturally sweet treat that also delivers nutritional benefits! The blend supports liver function, immune health, and digestion. Enjoy anytime for herbal benefits and a sweet treat!

DOSAGE: Add 2 to 4 tablespoons per cup of hot water or soda water.

INGREDIENTS

2 tablespoons dandelion root

2 tablespoons burdock root

2 tablespoons spearmint

2 sticks of reishi (approximately 2 tablespoons)

2 tablespoons sarsaparilla

2 tablespoons licorice

1 to 2 tablespoons fresh ginger (peeled, sliced and grated)

1 cinnamon stick

3 to 4 star anise pods

1 teaspoon black pepper

1 to 2 cups honey or cane sugar

INSTRUCTIONS: See syrup recipe on page 9.

HOW TO USE: Add syrup to hot water for sweet tea or add to soda water. Drop in a lemon slice!

TIP: Sugar preserves the syrup best, but honey is a good alternative. For less sweetness, use ¾ sweetener plus ¼ brandy for every cup of sugar. Less sweetener does mean a shorter shelf life.

Oxymels use half apple cider vinegar, half honey as a menstruum—tangy, sweet, and delicious! Experiment with any herbs.

DOSAGE: Take 1 to 4 tablespoons as desired.

INGREDIENTS

Equal parts of any of these herbs:

1 part nettles

1 part horsetail

1 part oat straw

1 part rose hip

1 part blackberry leaf

1 part dandelion root

1 part red clover buds

1 part hawthorn berries

1 part citrus peels (fresh or dried)

Apple cider vinegar

Honey

INSTRUCTIONS: Fill a pint or quart jar halfway with herbs. Add vinegar to half-full (measure if desired—8 ounces for pint jar). Fill the remainder of the jar with honey. Lid, shake, and then steep for 3 to 4 weeks in a cool, dark place. Shake regularly. Strain into a clean jar.

HOW TO USE: Take directly, add to soda water, or use to dress salads or vegetables!

TIP: Endless herb combinations are possible—get creative!

Grief

A syrup or cordial like this can be especially comforting during times of tenderness, if you are grieving or have low energy.

DOSAGE: Take 1 to 3 tablespoons, or drink to taste.

INGREDIENTS

6 tablespoons hawthorn berries

6 tablespoons hawthorn leaf and flower

1 cinnamon stick

3 tablespoons rose petals and/or buds

3 tablespoons rose hips

3 tablespoons hibiscus

1 tablespoon fresh grated ginger

1 to 2 cups of honey or cane sugar

¼ cup brandy (optional)

INSTRUCTIONS: Follow the syrup recipe on page 9.

HOW TO USE: Take directly by spoon in your mouth, mix it in hot water as a light tea, or add to soda water.

TIP: The sugar content preserves the syrup, though you can substitute honey (other alternatives such as coconut sugar don't work the same). If you avoid sugar or want less, remember that you're consuming very small amounts.

REMEDY: LINDEN OAT STRAW INFUSION FOR A BROKEN HEART

Simple infusions like this can be made with just about any herb. This infusion feels like a hug, calming your nervous system and soothing your heart.

DOSAGE: Drink 1 quart per day as needed.

INGREDIENTS

2 heaping tablespoons linden

2 heaping tablespoons oat straw

INSTRUCTIONS: Make this as a cold or hot infusion. For a cold infusion, place the herbs in a 1-quart jar (or equivalent) and cover with room temperature water. Let steep on the counter or in the fridge overnight; then strain and drink. For a hot infusion, steep the herbs in hot water for 15 to 30 minutes, and then strain and drink.

HOW TO USE: Drink as water throughout the day. Store unused portions in the refrigerator for up to 3 days.

TIP: This tea never turns bitter and has a mellow flavor, allowing for overnight steeping. If the linden becomes too mucilaginous (gooey), reduce steeping time. You'll discover your preferred infusion method.

REMEDY: SOOTHING SPIRIT HERBAL BATH

Herbal baths can be soothing to your soul! Make the tea first before adding to the bath—it's the only way to extract important constituents (putting herbs directly in the bath is messy too).

DOSAGE: Take 1 bath as needed.

INGREDIENTS

1 part calendula

1 part rose

1 part chamomile

INSTRUCTIONS: Add 1.5 cups of herbs to a ½ gallon-jar (or equivalent). Cover with boiling water. Steep covered for 15 minutes while filling your bathtub. Once the tea is ready, strain it directly into the bath.

HOW TO USE: Soak in the herbal bath and enjoy.

TIP: Bath water usually isn't hot enough to extract constituents properly, so always make the tea separately then add it to the bath!

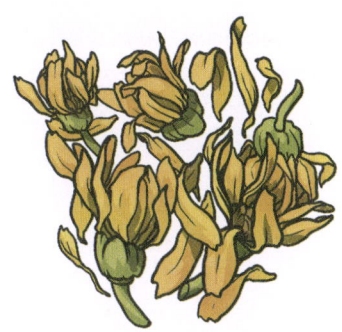

Hair Health

This recipe provides nutrients that promote healthy hair and skin!

DOSAGE: Drink 1 to 4 cups daily.

INGREDIENTS

2 parts nettles

2 parts oat buds or oat straw

1 part burdock root

1 part horsetail

1 part rosemary

½ part alfalfa

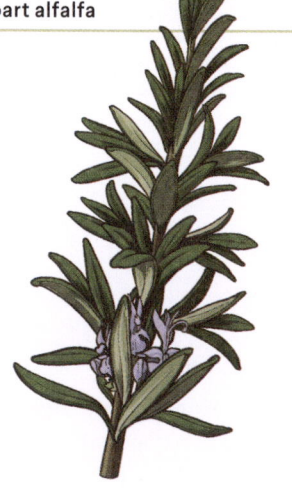

INSTRUCTIONS: Combine all ingredients and steep for 15 to 30 minutes, using 1 tablespoon of the herb mixture per cup of hot water. Strain and serve.

HOW TO USE: Make as a tea and drink warm.

TIP: Hair loss can be frightening when the cause is unknown. Common culprits include hormone imbalances, stress, or thyroid issues. Try relevant recipes from this book, and seek medical help if it worsens. Chinese herbal medicine often proves excellent for hair loss—consider consulting a Chinese herbalist.

REMEDY: FLAKY SCALP HAIR RINSE

Mild flaky scalp often results from seasonal dryness or product buildup (such as using the same shampoo for months). A vinegar rinse nourishes the hair and scalp, though the smell takes some adjustment!

DOSAGE: Use enough liquid to cover scalp and hair. Use after each shampoo for a couple of weeks.

INGREDIENTS

5 tablespoons calendula

3 tablespoons lemon peel (dried, if fresh use 4 to 5 tablespoons)

5 tablespoons burdock root

5 tablespoons rosemary

5 tablespoons horsetail

2 tablespoons thyme

1.5 cups of apple cider vinegar

Use essential oils of your choice for scent (try rose, geranium, lemongrass, chamomile, frankincense, or lavender)

INSTRUCTIONS: Fill a pint jar (or larger) with herbs, and add 1.5 to 2 cups of apple cider vinegar. Lid, label, and shake gently. Let it sit in a cool, dark place for 2 weeks. (You will need to check on the herbs after one day to make sure they are still covered. Add more vinegar to cover if needed.) Strain and pour it into a container. Add a few drops of essential oils if desired.

HOW TO USE: Before showering, dilute the mixture into a second bottle (1 part vinegar to 4 parts water). After shampooing and rinsing, pour the vinegar solution onto your scalp and work through your hair with your hands. Let it sit for a few minutes if time allows, and then rinse (use warm then cold water for extra shine). Use with every shampoo for a couple weeks to reduce flakiness, or whenever you feel product buildup.

TIP: The vinegar smell lingers briefly, but it does fade!

Hangover

I'm sorry, friend, but the only cure is time! Hangovers affect everyone differently. Start with a simple hydration tea—if that doesn't help, or if it worsens symptoms, check the Headache, Nausea, or Indigestion sections for additional remedies.

DOSAGE: Drink 1 cup to 1 quart of tea.

INGREDIENTS

Choose one herb: peppermint, ginger, or oat straw

INSTRUCTIONS: For nausea, try peppermint or ginger. Using 1 tablespoon of herb per cup of hot water, cover and steep for 15 minutes (if using fresh ginger, grate into your cup or simmer on the stove for 20 minutes). Strain and sip. For dehydration, try oat straw. Use 4 tablespoons in 1 quart of hot water, steep for a couple hours until cooled, and then sip throughout the day.

HOW TO USE: If the tea doesn't worsen symptoms, sip throughout the day whether it helps or has a neutral effect.

TIP: Herbs remineralize and rehydrate your body after alcohol's dehydrating effects.

Headaches

REMEDY: HEADACHE RELIEF TEA

Everything from headaches to migraines falls under "head pain" because diagnosis can be difficult. Head pain can be hormonal, digestive, tension-related, or some other migraine type. Try these remedies—if they don't work, test the herbs individually.

DOSAGE: Drink 1 cup as needed for head pain.

INGREDIENTS

1 part chamomile

1 part peppermint

1 part rosemary

INSTRUCTIONS: Combine all ingredients and steep for 10-15 minutes, using 1 tablespoon of the herb mixture per cup of hot water. Strain and serve.

HOW TO USE: Make as a tea and drink warm. Close your eyes and rest in a quiet, dark place to calm the pain.

TIP: Add feverfew to this blend if available—it has a long history of helping migraines!

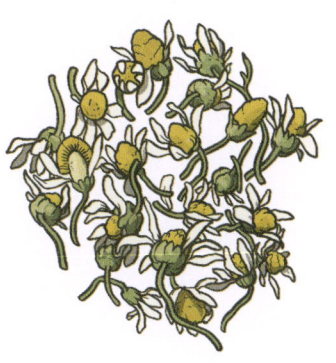

Willow bark provides amazing pain relief. Try this tincture
to ease your headache.

DOSAGE: Take 1 to 2 dropperfuls
and wait 30 minutes. If there is
no change, take another dose.
Try up to 4 times; then rest and
consider alternatives if the tincture doesn't provide relief.

INGREDIENTS

White willow bark

2 cups of 80 to 100 proof vodka

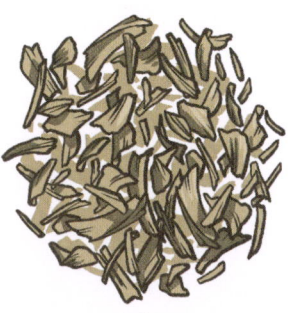

INSTRUCTIONS: Place the bark
in a pint jar, filling about halfway.
Cover with vodka. Lid, label, and
store in a cool, dry place for 3 to
4 weeks. Shake occasionally.
Strain and pour into a dropper
bottle to dose.

HOW TO USE: Use as needed,
either directly into your mouth
or in a shot glass with water.

TIP: This remedy works well
alongside teas that relax muscle
tension. Try the Stress or
Digestion section teas!

Heart Health

All the herbs in this blend support heart health, with hawthorn as the star! Drink daily and as often as desired.

DOSAGE: Drink 1 to 3 cups daily.

INGREDIENTS

2 parts hawthorn berries

2 parts hawthorn leaf and flower

1 part oat buds or oat straw

1 part lemon balm

1 part licorice

1 part linden

INSTRUCTIONS: Combine all ingredients and steep for 15 minutes or longer, using 2 tablespoons of the herb mixture per cup of hot water. Strain and serve.

HOW TO USE: Make as a tea and drink warm.

TIP: The licorice isn't just for flavor—it benefits the cardiovascular system. If you dislike licorice, remove it. The tea will be bland, so try adding peppermint.

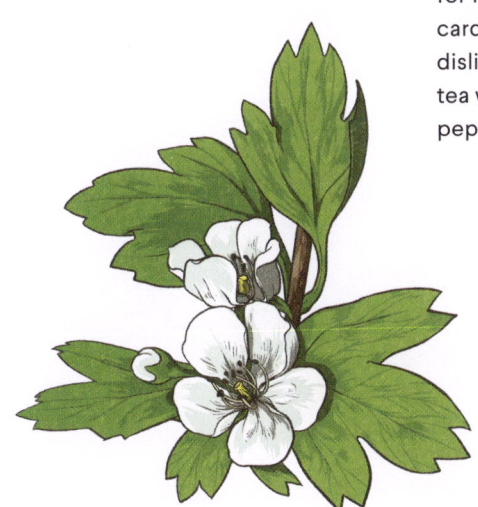

Hemorrhoids

For hemorrhoids, this wash soothes tissues and maintains smooth bowel movements. Daily sitz baths are recommended to keep bowels moving smoothly, and if desired, you can apply witch hazel topically (buy witch hazel pads or use cotton rounds dabbed with witch hazel toner and hold on the area). This wash works perfectly in your sitz bath.

DOSAGE: Perform 1 wash daily, preferably in the morning after a bowel movement.

INGREDIENTS

1 part chamomile

1 part calendula

A sprinkle of Epsom salt

INSTRUCTIONS: Prepare the tea. For a toilet sitz bath basin, make a 1-quart tea (¼ cup dried herbs to 1 quart of warm water). For a bathtub, use 1 cup dried herbs to ½ gallon of warm water. Steep the tea for 15 to 20 minutes, and then pour into your basin with Epsom salt. Cool if needed (add cool water to adjust the temperature). Sit for 10 minutes. Pat dry when finished.

HOW TO USE: Empty the basin after use and clean/dry it for the next use.

TIP: Drink the Easy Mover Tea while the tissues heal, keeping bowel movements smooth to prevent reopening wounds. Ensure adequate fiber, water, and exercise. Sitz bath basins fit over toilet seats and are available online. Epsom salts are optional. You can also add comfrey or oat buds.

Hormone Health

There are many approaches for regulating the menstrual cycle. Try drinking this tea for a couple of weeks monthly and note any changes.

DOSAGE: Drink 1 to 3 cups daily for 2 to 3 weeks per month until your cycle regulates.

INGREDIENTS

2 parts chaste tree berry (vitex)

2 parts dandelion root

2 parts sarsaparilla

1 part burdock

1 part spearmint

1 part ginger

1 part licorice

½ part cinnamon

INSTRUCTIONS: Combine all ingredients and steep for about 20 minutes, using 1 tablespoon of the herb mixture per cup of hot water. Strain and serve.

HOW TO USE: Make as a tea and drink warm.

TIP: Try making this as a decoction instead. Place herbs with 2 cups water in a saucepan and bring to a light simmer. Simmer on low for 15 to 20 minutes. Strain and serve. This extracts more medicinal qualities but tastes spicier.

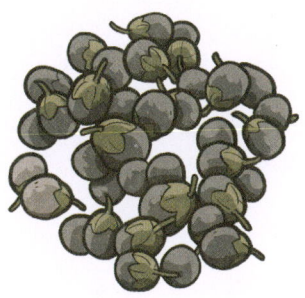

Hot Flashes

This remedy helps with hot flashes and heart palpitations during perimenopause.

DOSAGE: Take 1 to 2 dropperfuls 3 times daily as a tonic.

INGREDIENTS

4 tablespoons sage

4 tablespoons motherwort

2 tablespoons black cohosh

1.5 cups 80 to 100 proof vodka

INSTRUCTIONS: Add herbs to a pint (or larger) jar. Add the alcohol, lid, label, and let it sit for 3 to 4 weeks. Shake gently daily. Strain into a clean jar or dropper bottles.

HOW TO USE: Take a dose directly or in a shot glass of water.

TIP: Try this as a tea too, though it's very bitter—add spearmint, licorice, or peppermint.

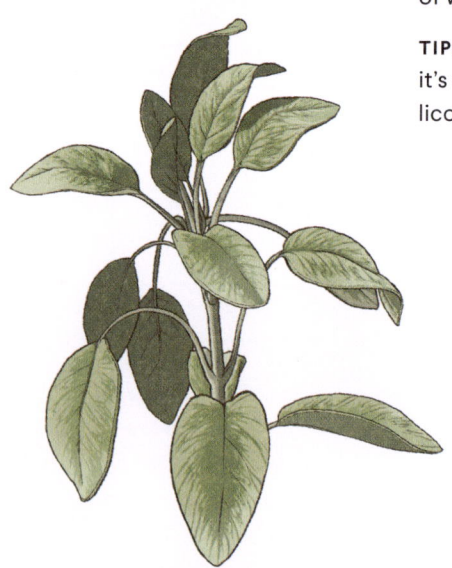

Immune Support

In Chinese medicine, getting sick more than three times yearly indicates a struggling immune system. This broth supports immunity if you have kids, fly frequently, teach, or encounter crowds often. Add these herbs to soup stocks and drink daily between illnesses (not while actively sick). Make chicken or herbal stock to drink daily, or incorporate them into foods such as oatmeal, soups, rice dishes, and stir-fries.

DOSAGE: Consume 1 cup of broth daily if possible or several times weekly (it can be chicken soup!).

INGREDIENTS

1 bay leaf

1 tablespoon calendula

1 tablespoon astragalus

2 to 3 sticks of reishi mushroom

1 tablespoon fenugreek

1 tablespoon dandelion root

1 teaspoon orange peel

1 teaspoon or stick of either wakame or kombu seaweed

INSTRUCTIONS: Add all ingredients to your bone broth in a slow cooker, or however you make chicken or beef broth. It adds a rich taste, especially in beef broth.

HOW TO USE: Drink the broth as tea, freeze portions, or refrigerate it. When needed, substitute in any recipe calling for water to add savory, immune-boosting nutrients. (Try making a savory oatmeal—it tastes amazing!)

TIP: Seaweeds aren't in our herb list, but they provide amazing health benefits. Their high mineral content supports our systems and is rare in Western diets. They enhance broth beautifully, but you can omit it if unavailable. The best choice is 1 stick of kombu.

Indigestion

Digestive bitters stimulate digestion and help break down fats after eating. Use them as appetite stimulants when needed and for overindulgence relief.

DOSAGE: Take a few drops to a dropperful 15 to 30 minutes before meals or directly after.

INGREDIENTS

1 part burdock root

1 part dandelion root

1 part dandelion leaf

1 part ginger (fresh or dried)

1 part yellow dock

1 part chamomile

2 cups of 80 to 100 proof vodka

INSTRUCTIONS: Place herbs in a pint jar in equal parts until half full. Cover with alcohol, lid, and shake gently. Label. Store in a cool, dry place for 3 to 4 weeks, shaking daily.

HOW TO USE: Put the drops directly in your mouth or under your tongue. It will be bitter!

TIP: The bitter flavors of the herbs stimulate digestive juices, so it is best to take it directly rather than in water. If you experience acid reflux from this, examine your diet or consult the Acid Reflux section.

Infertility

Infertility has many causes, but regulating your cycle always helps. This makes a great general women's tonic tea with a lovely flavor.

DOSAGE: Drink 1 to 3 cups daily for several weeks. Take breaks as desired, but regular use helps regulation.

INGREDIENTS

1 part lemon balm

1 part nettle

1 part spearmint

1 part raspberry leaf

½ part calendula

¼ part oat buds

¼ part stevia leaf

INSTRUCTIONS: Combine all ingredients and steep for 15 minutes, using 1 tablespoon of the herb mixture per cup of hot water. Strain and serve.

HOW TO USE: Make as a tea and drink it warm.

TIP: Omit the stevia leaf if you dislike the taste, but it adds a slightly sweet, lovely note to teas. Alternate with Women's Rooted Tea if desired.

Insomnia

If you struggle to wind down and fall asleep, the herbs in this formula will help you relax and prepare for bed.

DOSAGE: Drink 1 to 2 cups after dinner, with the latest consumed 30 to 60 minutes before bed.

INGREDIENTS

1 part skullcap

1 part oat buds

1 part chamomile

¼ part valerian

¼ part California poppy

INSTRUCTIONS: Combine all ingredients and steep for 15 minutes, using 1 tablespoon of the herb mixture per cup of hot water. Strain and serve.

HOW TO USE: It is best to drink one cup of tea a couple of hours before bed, and then sip some 1 hour before.

TIP: Omit the valerian root if the tea stops working. It's a temporary sleep aid, not for nightly dependence. Convert to tincture if tea causes nighttime bathroom trips.

REMEDY: GET BACK TO SLEEP TINCTURE

If falling asleep isn't the problem but waking in the night is, keep this tincture at your bedside with a small glass of water (or tincture glass).

DOSAGE: Take 1 dropperful as needed when you wake in the night.

INGREDIENTS

4 tablespoons passionflower

3 tablespoons ashwagandha

1 tablespoon lavender

1 cup vodka (80 to 100 proof)

INSTRUCTIONS: Place herbs in a pint jar. Pour vodka over the herbs, add the lid, shake, and label. Let it sit in a cool, dry place for 4 weeks. Strain into a clean jar. Fill a dropper bottle for bedside use.

HOW TO USE: Dose directly into your mouth or into a small shot glass with water.

TIP: You can also use this as a preventative. Take 1 to 2 dropperfuls 1 hour before bed and then another dose at bedtime.

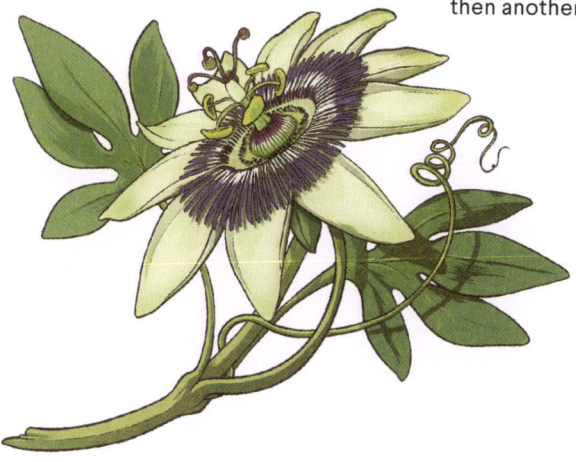

Irritability

Rose moves liver Qi in Chinese medicine—when Qi stagnates, we feel irritable, frustrated, and stuck. Rose smooths our energy and creates ease. Honey-sweetened cordials taste wonderful and deserve special cordial glasses!

DOSAGE: Take 1 to 2 tablespoons of cordial, as desired.

INGREDIENTS

½ cup dried rose petals (¾ cup fresh)

½ vanilla bean pod (chopped)

1.5 cups of brandy (more if using fresh rose)

¼ cup honey

2 tablespoons maple syrup

⅛ cup rose water

INSTRUCTIONS: Place rose petals and vanilla bean pod in a pint jar. Add brandy, ensuring the petals and bean pod are covered. Lid and label. Store in a cool, dark location for 4 weeks. Then strain through fine mesh. Discard herbs and add your sweetener blend (honey, maple syrup, and rose water work beautifully; customize as desired).

HOW TO USE: Best served in a cordial glass (like a tiny wine glass!). Otherwise pour into a shot glass or something enjoyable and sip. Grab your cordial, recline, take deep breaths (in through your nose and out through your mouth) to expel irritation. Sip and enjoy!

TIP: Don't use ornamental roses. Buy dried rose petals online (see herb supplier index). For fresh roses, *Rosa canina* (dog rose), *Rosa rugosa* (beach rose), or *Rosa multiflora* (wild rose) work wonderfully. When in doubt, use dried. Add ginger, cardamom, or cinnamon for complexity.

Jaw Pain

Jaw clenching and muscle tightness have become common issues. Acupuncture and manual therapy (massage or *gua sha*) help greatly. Heat and a soothing compress make an excellent remedy to try at home.

DOSAGE: Use 1 poultice per day as needed to soothe and relax your jaw muscles.

INGREDIENTS

2 tablespoons chamomile

1 tablespoons lavender

1 tablespoons rosemary

INSTRUCTIONS: Boil water. Place an open tea towel or handkerchief in a small bowl. Put the herbs in the towel's center and pour a couple of tablespoons of water onto them. You'll want warm-hot herbs that aren't soaking wet. Once the herbs are hydrated, grab the towel edges, pull them together, and hold (squeeze out excess water—it'll look like a little dumpling). If it's too dry, add another tablespoon of water and repeat.

HOW TO USE: Sit where you can recline. Place the poultice directly on your jaw, holding the towel with the herbs, and apply this little "dumpling" straight onto your jaw. Once it cools, add more hot water and repeat until you feel relief.

TIP: You can reuse these herbs several times. Leave the bowl with the herbs out to dry overnight. The next day add hot water and repeat.

Labor Support

Beginning at 36 weeks of pregnancy, you can start preparing for birth with the support of specific herbs. Daily raspberry leaf tea helps tone and prepare the uterus. Your baby won't arrive because you drink a cup of this tea, but if you're concerned, wait until you've reached 38 weeks or consult your doctor.

DOSAGE: Drink 1 to 4 cups daily.

INGREDIENTS

Raspberry leaf

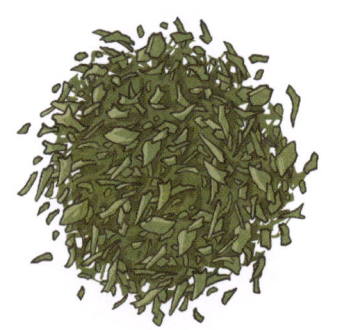

INSTRUCTIONS: Steep for 15 minutes, using 1 tablespoon of the raspberry leaf per cup of hot water. Strain and serve.

HOW TO USE: Make as a tea and drink warm.

TIP: To drink several cups daily, make one pot at a time! It's fine to drink if it cools down.

Liver Health

The liver manages metabolic waste in the system and masterfully detoxifies. It helps with hormonal imbalances and digestion. For acne, start by treating the liver.

DOSAGE: Take 2 dropperfuls 2 to 3 times daily for a medicinal dose. Reduce to twice daily if stomach upset occurs, or to 1 dropperful (about 30 drops) twice daily if issues persist. Titrate the dose to your sensitivity—some patients see results with just a few drops daily.

INGREDIENTS

1 part burdock root

1 part yellow dock

1 part red clover

1 part dandelion leaf

1 part dandelion root

2 cups of 80 to 100 proof vodka

INSTRUCTIONS: Place herbs in a pint jar until half full. Add vodka, filling it to the top. Lid, shake, and label. After 3 to 4 weeks, strain into a clean jar or dropper bottles.

HOW TO USE: The mixture is bitter. Take it directly or try this method: keep a small shot glass handy, fill it with water, add the tincture, and then drink.

TIP: Start slowly and adjust to your body's response.

REMEDY: CASTOR OIL PACK FOR LIVER DETOXING

Naturopathic doctors often prescribe castor oil packs for detoxing and internal medicine issues. These soothing treatments provide nice self-care while supporting liver health.

DOSAGE: Use 1 treatment daily for 1 to 2 weeks for gentle liver cleansing.

INGREDIENTS

Castor oil

INSTRUCTIONS: Prepare to relax for 30 to 45 minutes with a show or a book. Lift your shirt (wear something you don't mind staining) and apply 2 tablespoons of castor oil to your abdomen (apply it from a few inches below navel to your ribs, your liver sits under your right ribs, a few inches below your right nipple). To protect the towel from staining, after you've applied the castor oil, you can place plastic wrap over your abdomen, and then place the towel and put a heating pad on top. You can place the tea towel directly on your abdomen with the heating pad on top if you're not concerned with staining. Relax with the warmth for 30 to 45 minutes. When finished use a washcloth with warm water to wipe off the oil. The castor oil is sticky and stains—not all of it will come off, so wear an old T-shirt afterward.

HOW TO USE: Castor oil needs no refrigeration. Just clean up afterward!

TIP: Do this before bed and then sleep in an old T-shirt. Baking soda or OxiClean removes most stains from towels, but reusing the same towels works fine. For infused castor oil, follow the herbal oil recipe on page 9. Castor oil's thickness makes double boiler or infusion methods preferable to the alcohol-intermediary method. Try these infusions: ginger, St. John's wort, comfrey, calendula, or lavender.

Low Libido

Damiana has a reputation as an aphrodisiac, but it also nourishes the nervous system and acts as a mild antidepressant This cordial promotes happiness, and it may even get you in the mood!

DOSAGE: Take 1 to 2 tablespoons as needed.

INGREDIENTS

¼ cup damiana

1 vanilla bean chopped

2 tablespoons rose

2 tablespoons oat buds

1.5 cups brandy or vodka (80 to 100 proof)

¼ cup honey

⅛ rose water (optional)

INSTRUCTIONS: Place the herbs and vanilla bean in a pint jar. Add the alcohol, filling to about three-fourths full, and then add the honey. Lid, label, and shake gently. Let it sit in a cool dark place for 3 to 4 weeks, remembering to shake often. Strain and add rose water if desired.

HOW TO USE: Pour your cordial into a cordial glass—perhaps something you and partner can enjoy together 30 to 60 minutes before your date. Sip and let yourself relax!

TIP: This recipe adds honey during steeping, but experiment with adding it afterward instead. The herbs absorb some honey, so adding it after creates a sweeter result.

Lung Health

After a respiratory illness—or following exposure to smoke or other lung-compromising conditions—this tea is a great way to nourish lung tissue.

DOSAGE: Drink 1 to 3 cups daily as needed.

INGREDIENTS

1 part mullein

1 part peppermint

½ part marshmallow leaf

½ part marshmallow root

½ part fennel

½ part licorice

INSTRUCTIONS: Combine all ingredients and steep for 15 minutes, using 1 tablespoon of the herb mixture per cup of hot water. Strain and serve.

HOW TO USE: Make as a tea and drink warm.

TIP: Add honey to nourish the throat as well.

Lymph Support

If your lymphatic system feels sluggish, this tea may offer support. It contains diuretic herbs, so be sure to stay well hydrated by drinking plenty of water!

DOSAGE: Drink 1 to 3 cups daily as needed.

INGREDIENTS

1 part mullein

1 part calendula

½ part cleavers

½ part dandelion root

¼ part licorice

INSTRUCTIONS: Combine all ingredients and steep for 10 minutes, using 1 tablespoon of the herb mixture per cup of hot water. Strain and serve.

HOW TO USE: Make as a tea and drink warm.

TIP: If you dislike licorice, substitute peppermint, spearmint, or another tasty herb. For extra diuretic power, you can add plantain.

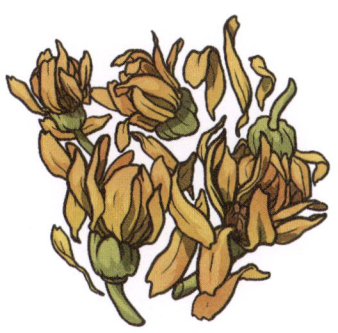

Nausea

Whether nauseous from a heavy meal or first trimester pregnancy, this soothing tea can help calm your stomach.

DOSAGE: Drink 1 cup as needed for nausea.

INGREDIENTS

1 part ginger

1 part marshmallow root

1 part spearmint

INSTRUCTIONS: Combine all ingredients and steep for 10 to 15 minutes, using 1 tablespoon of the herb mixture per cup of hot water. Strain and serve.

HOW TO USE: Make as a tea and sip when warm.

TIP: When nauseous, adding anything to your stomach can feel challenging—especially during pregnancy's first trimester. Make the tea and take small sips. It's fine if drinking takes some time.

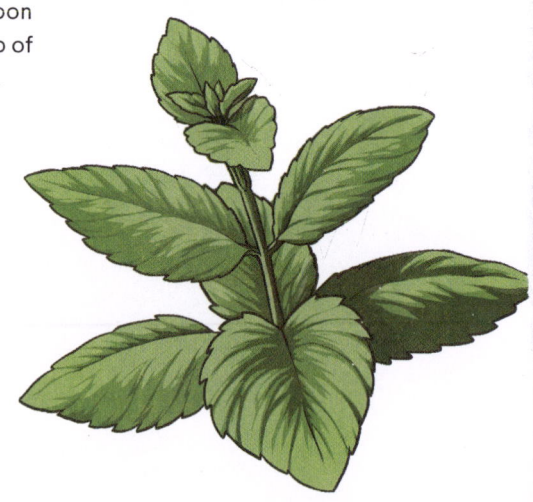

Night Sweats

This tincture is a modification of the hot flash tincture formula. While it may not stop hot flashes completely, it works to balance the system. If this doesn't provide relief, try the Cool Me Down Hot Flash Tincture instead.

DOSAGE: Take 1 to 2 dropperfuls 3 times daily as a tonic.

INGREDIENTS

2 tablespoons black cohosh

4 tablespoons sage

3 tablespoons red clover blossoms

1 tablespoon licorice

1.5 cups 80 to 100 proof vodka

INSTRUCTIONS: Prepare your tincture by adding the herbs to a pint jar (or larger), filling halfway. Cover with alcohol. Lid, label, and let sit for 3 to 4 weeks. Shake gently daily or every other day.

HOW TO USE: Take a dose directly or in a shot glass of water.

TIP: During perimenopause and menopause, adding good fats and oils such as flaxseed (seeds or oil) or evening primrose oil into your diet is crucial. Alcohol can significantly increase body heat. Discuss additional nutritional support with your doctor.

Nursing Mothers

REMEDY: MOTHER'S NURSING BLEND

Many patients have loved this blend while breastfeeding. It's called a nursing blend because the herbs support milk production. Even if you don't need increased production or choose not to breastfeed, this is an excellent postpartum tonic for hormone regulation, uterine tonification, and new mother nourishment.

DOSAGE: Drink 3 cups daily as needed during postpartum.

INGREDIENTS

1 part raspberry leaf

1 part oat straw

1 part fenugreek

1 part blessed thistle

½ part nettles

½ part rose hips

¼ part red clover blossoms

¼ part orange peel

INSTRUCTIONS: Combine all ingredients and steep for 15 minutes, using 1 tablespoon of the herb mixture per cup of hot water. Strain and serve.

HOW TO USE: Make as a tea and drink warm.

TIP: If you make extra, refrigerate and save for the next dose. Use it within 3 days.

Pain

When in pain, attack it comprehensively! This tea contains antispasmodics to soothe nerves and reduce muscle spasming. For extra relief, take the Willow Bark Tincture for Head Pain (page 80) and apply the St. John's Wort Sore Muscle Rub on the next page to aching areas. An herbal bath or foot soak also provides comfort.

DOSAGE: Drink 1 to 3 cups as needed for pain.

INGREDIENTS

1 part chamomile

1 part skullcap

1 part oat buds or oat straw

1 part ginger

½ part California poppy

½ part cassia chips

INSTRUCTIONS: Combine all ingredients and steep for 15 minutes, using 1 tablespoon of the herb mixture per cup of hot water. Strain and serve.

HOW TO USE: Make as a tea and drink warm.

TIP: Unless your injury is new and still red, hot, or inflamed, heat is your friend. Use a heating pad or hot water bottle while sipping this tea.

REMEDY: ST. JOHN'S WORT SORE MUSCLE RUB

As an acupuncturist who specializes in pain management, I love herbal topicals and swap between a few of them. Cayenne—a warming, circulatory herb—soothes pain and sore muscles.

DOSAGE: Apply as often as needed.

INGREDIENTS

4 ounces St. John's Wort Oil (find the recipe below or buy premade)

2 teaspoons cayenne pepper powder

2 tablespoons of beeswax pastilles

Optional: essential oils (rosemary, cypress, lavender, or chamomile for scent/pain relief)

INSTRUCTIONS: Combine oil and cayenne in a double boiler (or use a bowl and thick glass jar inside a saucepan with simmering water—choose the glass carefully to prevent breaking). Heat oil slightly and then cool. Gently reheat (twice-heating releases more pain-relieving constituents from cayenne). Remove from heat and infuse for 24 hours. Strain using a cheesecloth over a strainer and measuring cup, squeezing out the remaining oil. Using the double boiler again, reheat the remaining oil, add beeswax pastilles, and stir with a chopstick until melted. Remove from heat immediately. Add essential oils if desired (20 to 40 drops) and stir. Pour into tins or small jars (I use two 2-ounce jars). Cool completely before lidding.

HOW TO USE: Apply with fingers to sore muscles as needed.

TIP: Don't touch your eyes after using this! Salves last for months to years if kept in a cool, dry place and lidded.

REMEDY: ST. JOHN'S WORT OIL

Fresh St. John's wort flowers found in springtime (around early June), make excellent massage oil for sore muscles or as a base for the preceding muscle rub.

DOSAGE: Use as often as desired.

INGREDIENTS

Fresh St. John's wort flower

Olive oil (or grapeseed, almond, or apricot)

INSTRUCTIONS: Gather enough flowers to fill a small jar (8 to 16 ounces) almost completely. Start small (8-ounce jar) since finding enough fresh flowers can be challenging. Lay the flowers on paper towels, in a basket, or on newspaper for a few hours to overnight for a slight wilting. Then place the flowers in the jar and cover with oil. Lid, label, and shake gently. Place the jar in a sunny window for sun infusion, shaking daily. Infuse for 2 to 4 weeks (watch for water to avoid spoiling). When ready the oil turns deep red. Strain through a fine sieve with cheesecloth over Pyrex, squeezing the flowers to extract the remaining Hypericum. Store in a chosen bottle in a cool, dry place.

HOW TO USE: Use as a massage oil for tired feet, back, neck—anywhere! It works as a general body oil too. You can convert this to a salve recipe as described in the Making Herbal Medicine section.

TIP: Harvest St. John's wort when the flowers haven't quite opened, sticking mostly to the flower tops. Dried St. John's wort doesn't work as well in this recipe.

PMS (Premenstrual Syndrome)

Common PMS symptoms include mood changes, irritability, bloating, cramps, tender breasts, and depression. Try this tea first, then explore the sections matching your specific symptoms if needed.

DOSAGE: Drink 1 to 3 cups daily as needed for PMS symptoms.

INGREDIENTS

2 parts raspberry leaf

2 parts oat buds or oat straw

1 part lemon balm or spearmint

1 part lemon verbena

½ part rose

INSTRUCTIONS: Combine all ingredients and steep for 10 minutes, using 1 tablespoon of the herb mixture per cup of hot water. Strain and serve.

HOW TO USE: Make as a tea and serve warm.

TIP: For irritability, check the Irritability section too. Regular 20- to 30-minute walks can help move and soothe liver Qi in Chinese medicine—see if this creates positive changes.

Pregnancy

Always try this remedy first for pregnancy nausea.

DOSAGE: Drink 1 cup as needed.

INGREDIENTS

1-inch knob of fresh ginger root
(peeled and sliced into discs)

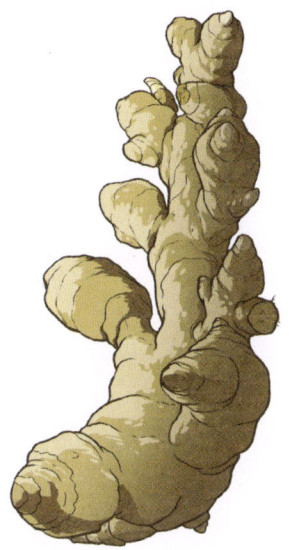

INSTRUCTIONS: Cut the ginger root into small discs and place in a saucepan. Cover with 1 to 2 cups of water (measure using your mug plus extra). Bring to a simmer, and then reduce heat to low for 20 minutes. Strain and serve.

HOW TO USE: Make as a tea and sip.

TIP: If smells make it difficult to ingest anything, let the tea cool to reduce the scent, then sip slowly over time. Small sips work fine.

Postpartum Support

See Anxiety (page 29) or Depression (page 54) sections for postpartum mood changes. For significant blood loss during birth or postpartum hair loss, make the Herbal Iron Syrup from the Anemia section. See the Nursing Mothers section for milk production support. Try Women's Rooted Tea for hormonal rebalancing.

REMEDY: POSTPARTUM SITZ BATH

After birth, perineal discomfort responds well to this soothing, healing sitz bath.

DOSAGE: Take 1 to 2 sitz baths daily.

INGREDIENTS

1 part calendula

1 part comfrey

1 part rose

1 part rosemary

Sitz bath basin or tub

INSTRUCTIONS: Combine ingredients in bowl or jar (1 ounce of each herb provides multiple baths). Steep ¼ cup of the herb mixture in 1 quart water from 30 minutes to overnight (shorter steeping works fine—since you're not drinking it, taste doesn't matter). Strain the tea into your sitz bath basin (a bathtub requires a larger batch—approximately 1 cup herb per ½ gallon of water). For overnight steeping, warm the tea slightly before use.

HOW TO USE: Pour the tea into the basin, and then sit and soak for 10 minutes. Pat yourself dry gently afterward.

TIP: Sitz bath basins over toilet seats or large floor basins work best—bathtubs require excessive liquid.

REMEDY: AFTER BIRTH REBALANCE TEA

After birth, hormones need rebalancing. Customize this recipe based on your symptoms.

DOSAGE: Drink 1 to 3 cups daily.

INGREDIENTS

Base blend

1 part nettles

1 part raspberry leaf

1 part calendula

Additional herbs

½ part St. John's wort and/or rose for depression

½ part motherwort for anxiety

½ part chaste tree berry (vitex) for hormone support

½ part ginger for cramping or digestive discomfort

INSTRUCTIONS: Combine the base blend (1 tablespoon each) with ½ tablespoon of any additional herbs. For one cup, mix 1 to 2 tablespoons dried herb total. Steep for 10 minutes, strain, and serve.

HOW TO USE: Make as a tea and drink warm.

TIP: Check the Anemia, Anxiety, Depression, Hormone Health, and Nursing Mothers sections for additional support.

Psoriasis

REMEDY: PSORIASIS RELIEF TEA

Psoriasis treatment often starts with liver support—this blend provides gentle liver support and detoxification. If you can identify your triggers, explore relevant book sections for those remedies (stress, sleep, etc.).

DOSAGE: Drink 3 cups daily as needed.

INGREDIENTS

1 part burdock

1 part sarsaparilla

1 part cleavers

1 part yellow dock

INSTRUCTIONS: Combine all ingredients and steep for 10 to 15 minutes, using 1 tablespoon of the herb mixture per cup of hot water. Strain and serve.

HOW TO USE: Make as a tea and drink warm.

TIP: This tea tastes quite bitter—persevere! Check the Skin Care section for a helpful salve recipe.

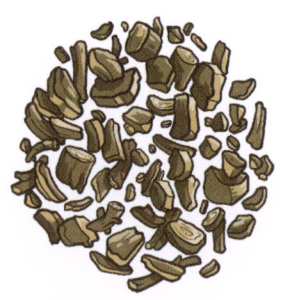

Rashes

When skin becomes irritated and develops a rash, use this soothing calendula wash for cooling relief.

DOSAGE: Use at least once daily.

INGREDIENTS

Calendula

Aloe gel (optional)

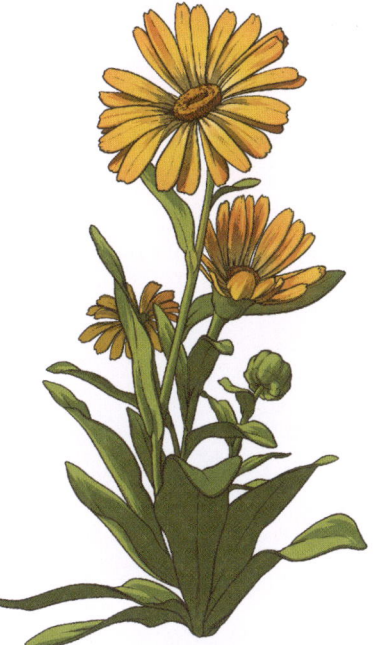

INSTRUCTIONS: Make a strong calendula tea using 2 tablespoons of calendula per cup of hot water (use a cup, French press, or pot). Steep for 15 to 30 minutes or longer, and then refrigerate.

HOW TO USE: Once cool, sit where you can comfortably apply a wet towel to the rash area. Dip the tea towel in the cool tea and place on the irritated area for 15 to 30 minutes. Re-wet the towel as needed (this gets messy—place extra towels underneath).

TIP: Add 1 to 2 tablespoons of aloe gel to the tea water if desired. For unexplained red, itchy, inflamed skin, consult your doctor or dermatologist, especially if it is spreading.

Restless Legs

Restless legs have various causes, but nourishing the system with magnesium and mineral-rich, antispasmodic herbs can help calm nerves and muscles. Oat buds prove especially helpful for the nervous system or nerve-related issues, and they are packed full of magnesium!

DOSAGE: Drink 1 to 3 cups daily as needed.

INGREDIENTS

2 parts milky oats or oat straw

1 part peppermint

1 part nettles

¼ part licorice (or more if desired)

INSTRUCTIONS: Combine all ingredients and steep for 10 to 15 minutes, using 1 tablespoon of the herb mixture per cup of hot water. Strain and serve.

HOW TO USE: Make as a tea and drink warm.

TIP: If you omit the licorice, steep considerably longer for a full extraction.

Seasonal Affective Disorder

REMEDY: LET THE SUN IN TEA

This tea provides warmth and brightens mood! Nourishing your system with herbs through the winter creates a beneficial practice for navigating darker months.

DOSAGE: Drink 1 to 3 cups daily as desired.

INGREDIENTS

1 part tulsi

1 part damiana

½ part rose

½ part lavender

INSTRUCTIONS: Combine all ingredients and steep for 10 minutes, using 1 tablespoon of the herb mixture per cup of hot water. Strain and serve.

HOW TO USE: Make as a tea and drink warm.

TIP: This is great with honey!

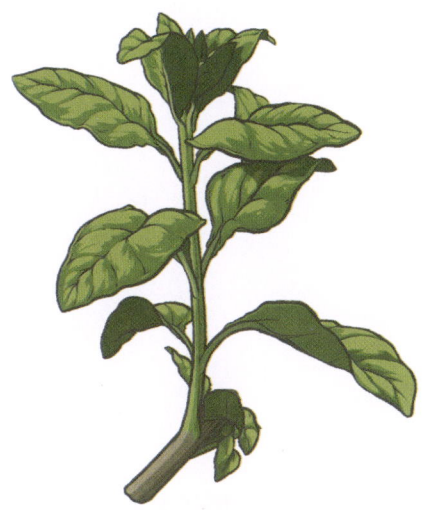

Skin Care

Herbal facial steams feel wonderful and benefit skin through improved circulation, offering beautiful results.

DOSAGE: Steam as desired—weekly works well, but not daily. Reduce if breakouts occur or skin worsens.

INGREDIENTS

2 parts calendula

2 parts lavender

2 parts rose

1 part peppermint

1 part raspberry leaf

1 part white willow bark

INSTRUCTIONS: Mix the herbal blend in a separate container (using tablespoons creates extra for later). Add 2 to 3 tablespoons of the herb blend to a large bowl. Boil water and pour 2 cups over the herbs (no need to fill the bowl since you'll position your face above it). Swirl the herbs to ensure water coverage. Position your face over the bowl and wrap a towel around your head and the bowl (wait if it's too hot to avoid burns). Set a timer for 5 to 10 minutes, ensuring the towel can trap vapors. Breathe the steam in and feel it nourishing your skin! Afterward pat your face dry. Cool the herbs before straining and discarding (use a mesh strainer in your sink drain).

HOW TO USE: Follow instructions above.

TIP: Customize the blend based on your skin's needs.

REMEDY: FLORAL HERBAL TONER

This makes a lovely witch hazel toner replacement or hydrating facial spritz.

DOSAGE: Use as needed.

INGREDIENTS

5 tablespoons calendula

4 tablespoons lavender

4 tablespoons lemon balm

4 tablespoons chamomile

4 tablespoons roses

3 tablespoons comfrey

1 tablespoon lemon peel (dried or fresh)

1 tablespoon rosemary

1 tablespoon elderflower

2 cups witch hazel

INSTRUCTIONS: Place the herbs in a pint jar and cover with witch hazel. For the rose water addition, use ¾ witch hazel and ¼ rose water. Lid and label. Place in a window for two weeks for a gentle heat extraction from the sun. Strain into a bottle (glass or spray bottle preferred).

HOW TO USE: After cleansing, spray directly on your skin or apply gently with a cotton pad. Spray your face directly when needing extra hydration.

TIP: For more floral scent, substitute some witch hazel for the rose water. If it is too strong, halve the herb recipe or add more liquid.

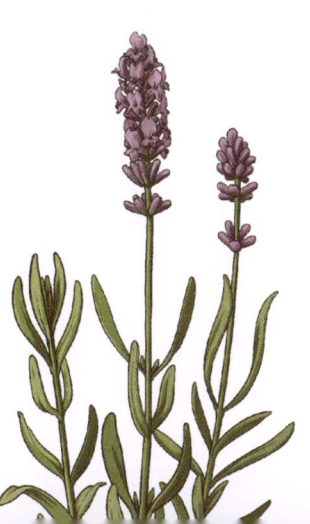

REMEDY: CALENDULA COMFREY SKIN SALVE

Every herbalist keeps some version of this salve handy. Perfect for dry skin, minor injuries, irritations—or anything that needs soothing. This salve contains demulcent herbs such as plantain and calendula, plus wound-healing comfrey. This recipe has two parts: making the herbal oil and then creating the salve with beeswax (vegan versions use carnauba wax but results vary).

DOSAGE: Use a pea-sized amount as needed.

INGREDIENTS

⅔ cup dried calendula

⅔ cup dried comfrey

⅔ cup dried plantain

1.5 cups olive oil

1.5 to 2 teaspoons 80 to 100 proof vodka

2 tablespoons beeswax pastilles

INSTRUCTIONS:

PART 1: Make herbal oil following the alcohol-intermediary method on page 10.

PART 2: Strain the oil through a sieve with cheesecloth, squeezing out the remainder. Measure 1 cup of infused oil and add it to a double boiler over low-medium heat. Add beeswax and heat until melted (stir with a chopstick). Remove from heat and add essential oils if desired (20 to 40 drops). Pour immediately into tins or jars. Let stand, uncovered, to cool and harden before lidding.

HOW TO USE: Rub on skin as needed to hydrate and heal.

TIP: Single-herb salves work fine too—omit any herbs as desired.

Sprains & Strains

REMEDY: SORE MUSCLE COMPRESS

While heating pads provide comfort for strained muscles, herbal compresses offer next-level relief!

DOSAGE: Use up to 3 compresses daily.

INGREDIENTS

1 part blackberry leaf

1 part yarrow

1 part comfrey

Small cloth

INSTRUCTIONS: Mix herbs in a small bowl, using ½ cup of herbs per quart of hot water. This can also be made in a ½ gallon-jar if more water is needed for a larger area (requiring I cup of herbs). Pour boiling water over the herbs and cover for 15 minutes. Strain into a bowl or clean jar.

HOW TO USE: Soak a cloth in the tea, wring it out, and place it on the injury. Leave on for 15 minutes or until it needs rewarming.

TIP: Rose or chamomile make lovely additions! This also works as a poultice.

Stress

This tea melts stress away! Full of antispasmodics, it will both calm and relax you.

DOSAGE: Drink as often as needed throughout the day to feel calm.

INGREDIENTS

2 parts chamomile

1 part passionflower

1 part skullcap

1 part oat straw

½ part lavender

INSTRUCTIONS: Combine all ingredients and steep for 8 to 10 minutes, using 1 tablespoon of the herb mixture per cup of hot water. Strain and serve.

HOW TO USE: Make as a tea and drink warm. This effective blend tastes a little bland, so consider adding honey. Swap out the lavender for lemon verbena if you prefer that flavor profile.

TIP: Pair this with a foot bath or herbal compress/poultice on your neck.

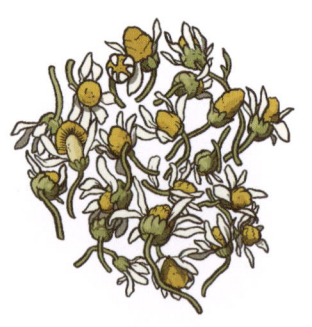

REMEDY: STRESS LESS HERBAL CHAI

For frequent stress, consider daily adrenal support. This caffeine-free chai contains adaptogenic herbs that help your body combat stress over time.

DOSAGE: Drink 1 to 3 cups daily as needed for energy.

INGREDIENTS

1.5 teaspoons cassia chips

1 teaspoon ginger (fresh or dried)

1 teaspoon ashwagandha

1 teaspoon astragalus (or 1 stick)

½ teaspoon licorice

½ teaspoon cloves

5 green cardamom pods

¼ teaspoon fennel

2 star anise pods

INSTRUCTIONS: Place all ingredients in a saucepan with 3 to 4 cups of water and bring to a simmer. Cook on low simmer (not boiling) for about 30 minutes. Strain and serve.

HOW TO USE: Drink plain or add milk and a sweetener of your choice (cream and honey or maple syrup work wonderfully).

TIP: Green cardamom pods and fresh ginger create the best flavor! Green cardamom offers a lovely complexity with a hint of mint. Black cardamom or powder substitutes work too. Dried ginger adds extra spice. Astragalus comes cut or in long tongue-depressor-like sticks—use about 1 teaspoon equivalent.

Sore Throat

REMEDY: SORE THROAT SOOTHER

Licorice provides powerful antibacterial and antiviral properties that help fight infection while soothing the throat. Its mucilaginous properties, combined with marshmallow, coat the throat effectively.

DOSAGE: Drink 1 cup as needed.

INGREDIENTS

1 part licorice root

1 part marshmallow root

1 part peppermint

½ part marshmallow leaf

INSTRUCTIONS: Combine all ingredients and steep for 15 minutes, using 1 tablespoon of the herb mixture per cup of hot water. Strain and serve.

HOW TO USE: Make as a tea and drink warm. If you add honey, try holding a sip in the back of your throat briefly for a coating effect.

TIP: If licorice isn't appealing, try the classic saltwater gargle! Add about 1 teaspoon salt to warm water, and gargle each sip several times until the cup empties.

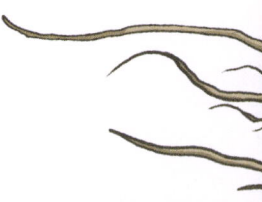

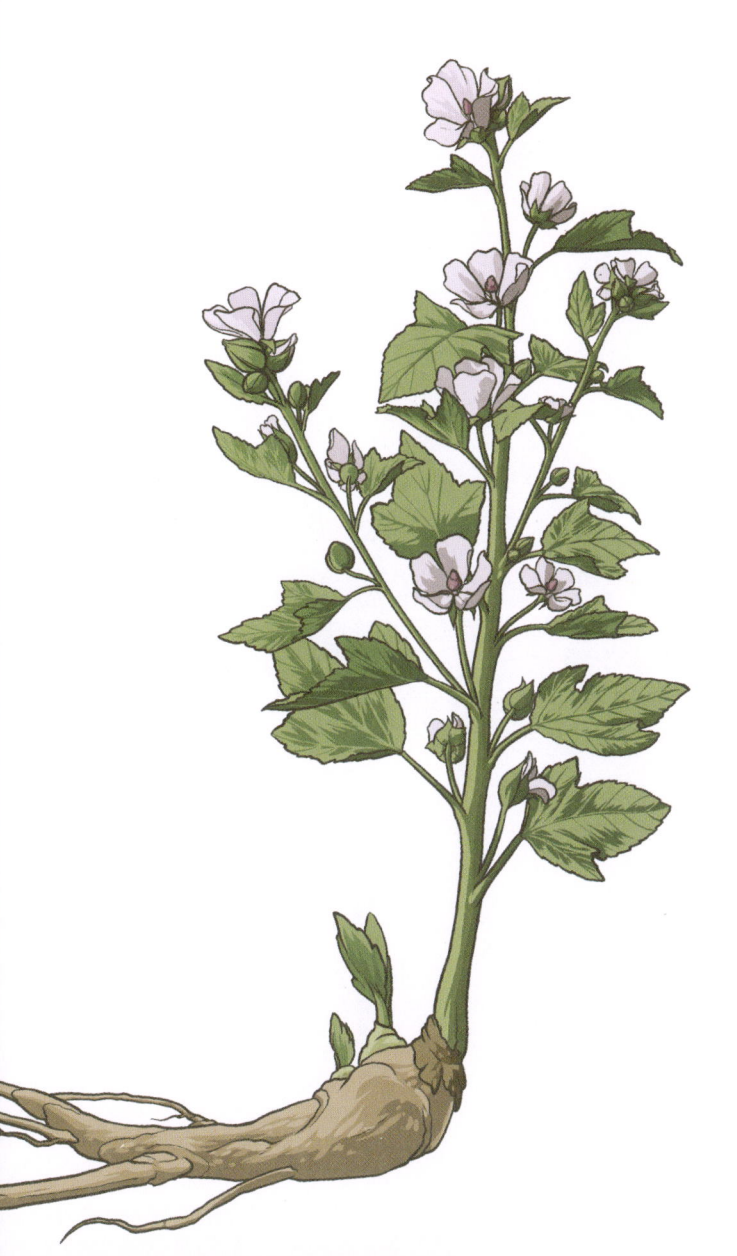

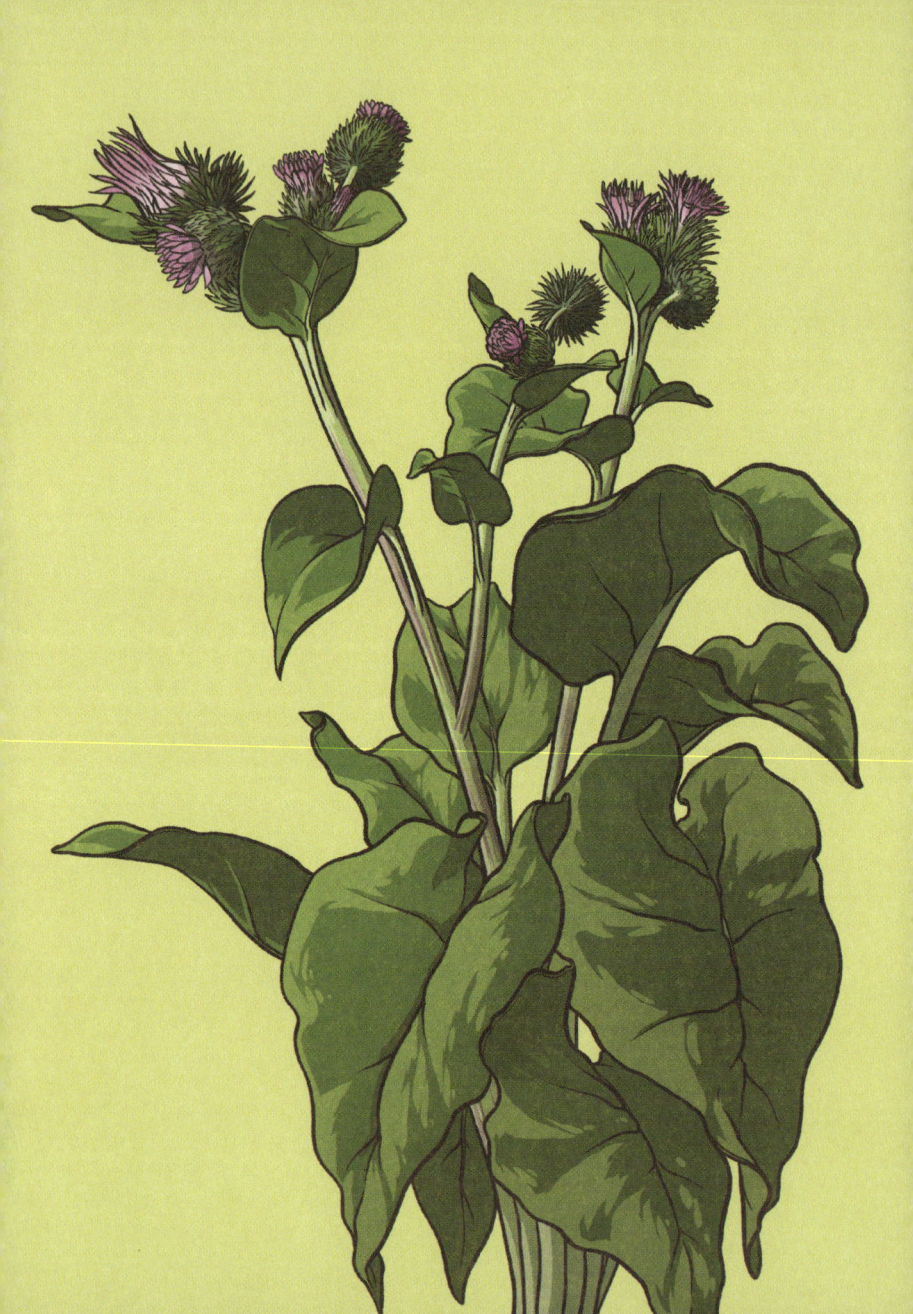

PART 3

Common Herbs

Herb Profiles

This section outlines the profiles of all the herbs used in this book, including taste, flavor, organ affinities (organs or body areas where the herb works best), folklore, and other useful information. Herbalists often write detailed monographs—essays about plants—and one plant's information could fill an entire booklet. These profiles offer essential snippets to help you get acquainted with these botanical allies. The medicinal actions described come from personal and clinical experience, with citations for information from other sources (especially chemical and nutritional aspects) and insights from respected herbalist colleagues.

Regarding safety considerations—herb and drug interactions remain understudied. The primary reference here is Francis Brinker's *Herb Contraindications and Drug Interactions*, one of the few publications with linked studies providing clinical perspectives on how modern drugs and herbs interact. Many herbs are contraindicated during pregnancy. Those with a history of miscarriage or complicated medical conditions should work closely with qualified healthcare practitioners who can safely guide herbal medicine use during pregnancy (naturopaths, acupuncturists, and herbalists—ask about their qualifications and experience).

Remember: herbs are plants, plants are food, and most low doses are safe for many people (drinking tea a few times weekly or taking occasional low-dose tinctures). However if you take life-saving medications, protecting their effectiveness is paramount.

Note: herbal medicine terms are defined on first use, then used freely throughout.

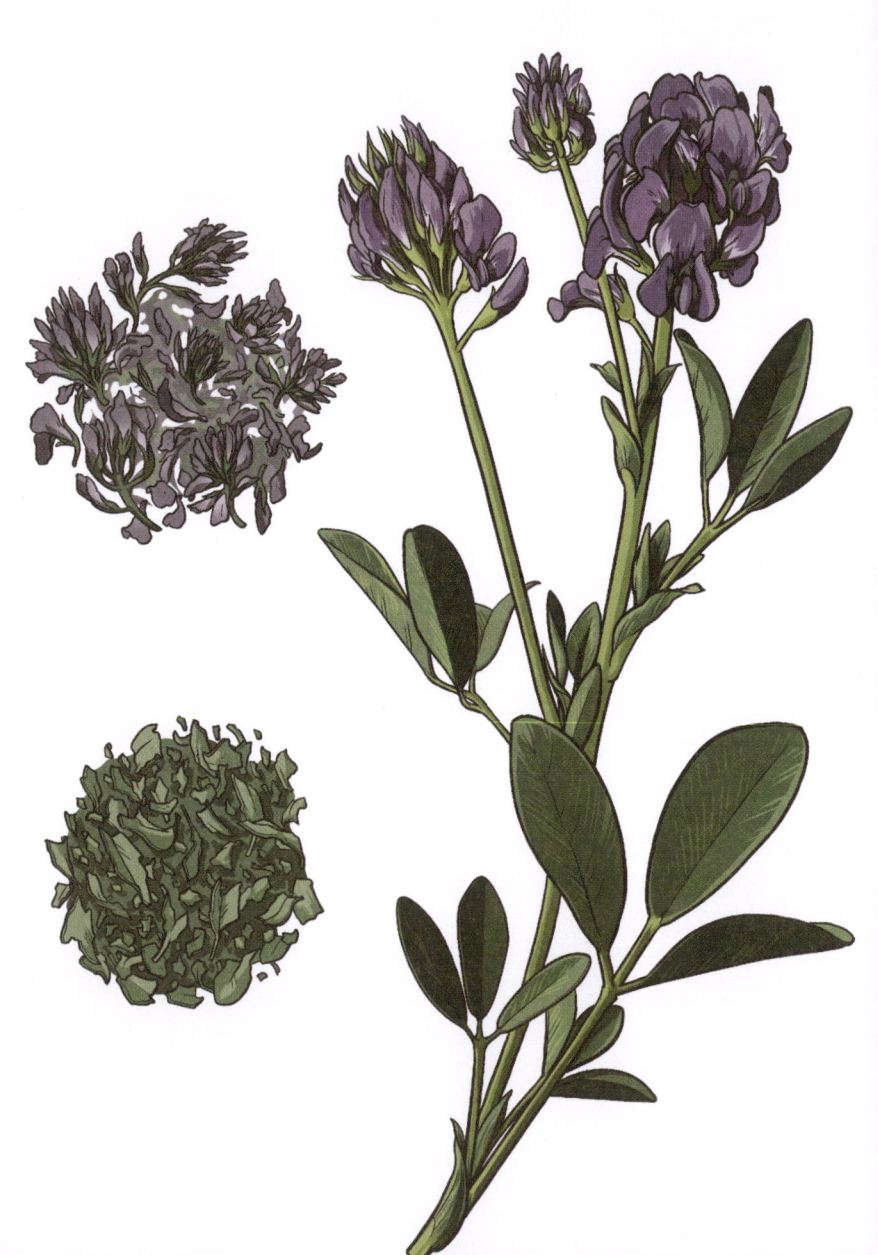

1

Alfalfa

Medicago sativa

Other name(s): lucerne, purple medic, buffalo grass

Alfalfa is sweet, cool, moisturizing, and very yin-nourishing for organs and tissues. Nutritious and anti-inflammatory, it supports breastfeeding mothers beautifully. As a legume (you know it as grocery store sprouts), it contains phytoestrogenic compounds. It may help lower cholesterol. Rich in trace minerals (calcium, magnesium, iron, potassium, riboflavin, and niacin), alfalfa benefits those with anemia, fatigue, and poor digestion, making it an excellent postpartum aid for blood loss and hormone regulation. It is best taken as a tea, tablet, powder, or tincture.

PARTS USED: aerial parts (all structures above ground: flowers, leaves, stems, stalks, and seeds)

MEDICINAL USES: anti-inflammatory, diuretic, nutritive, phytoestrogenic (plant compounds mimicking estrogen), support of milk production

SAFETY CONSIDERATIONS: Use cautiously in pregnancy due to uterine stimulant action and phytoestrogenic qualities. This may reduce the effectiveness of blood-thinning medications such as Warfarin due to its vitamin K content. Those with lupus erythematosus should avoid long-term use.

REMEDIES: Herbal Iron Syrup, Cholesterol Helper Tea, Bone Strength Tea, Shiny Happy Hair Tea

TIP: Start with small amounts to assess your body's response.

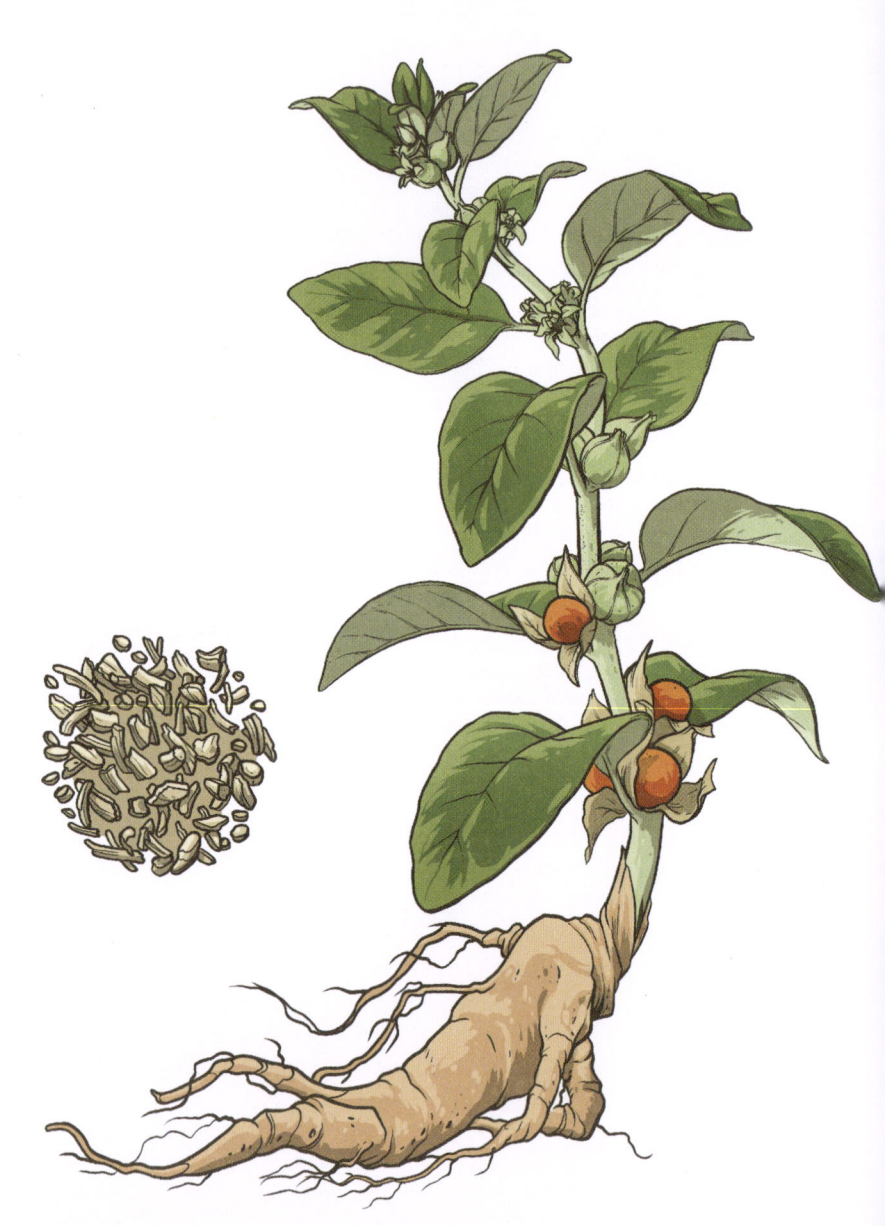

2

Ashwagandha

Withania somnifera
Other name(s): winter cherry

Ashwagandha is warm, bitter, astringent, and sweet—an herb from India first introduced by herbal teacher Karta Purkh Singh Khalsa. This nightshade family member (*Solanaceae*) provides relaxation and, over time, rejuvenation. Years of clinical use show it helps with nervous exhaustion, sexual debilitation, memory loss, and insomnia. In urban settings, it's commonly prescribed for those exhausted and agitated from stress who need rejuvenation, strength, and vitality. Properties include sedative, tonic, anti-inflammatory, and immune-balancing effects. As a tonic herb or adaptogen, it may take weeks to months to achieve full effects. For sleep it works better as a long-term tonic than an immediate sedative, tonifying sleep patterns over time. Dr. Sharol Tilgner notes it can increase thyroid (T4) levels in mice and humans. It is best taken as a decoction, powder, or tincture.

PARTS USED: root

MEDICINAL USES: nervous or stress-related exhaustion, impotence, age-related cognitive function, anti-inflammatory. It is helpful for staying asleep when taken long-term (not for falling asleep initially).

SAFETY CONSIDERATIONS: It is contraindicated during pregnancy. Due to its sedative effects, use caution with barbiturates and sleep aids such as benzodiazepines.

REMEDIES: Get Back to Sleep Tincture, Stress Less Herbal Chai

TIP: Occasionally this herb energizes rather than calms. Start with the smallest dosage first.

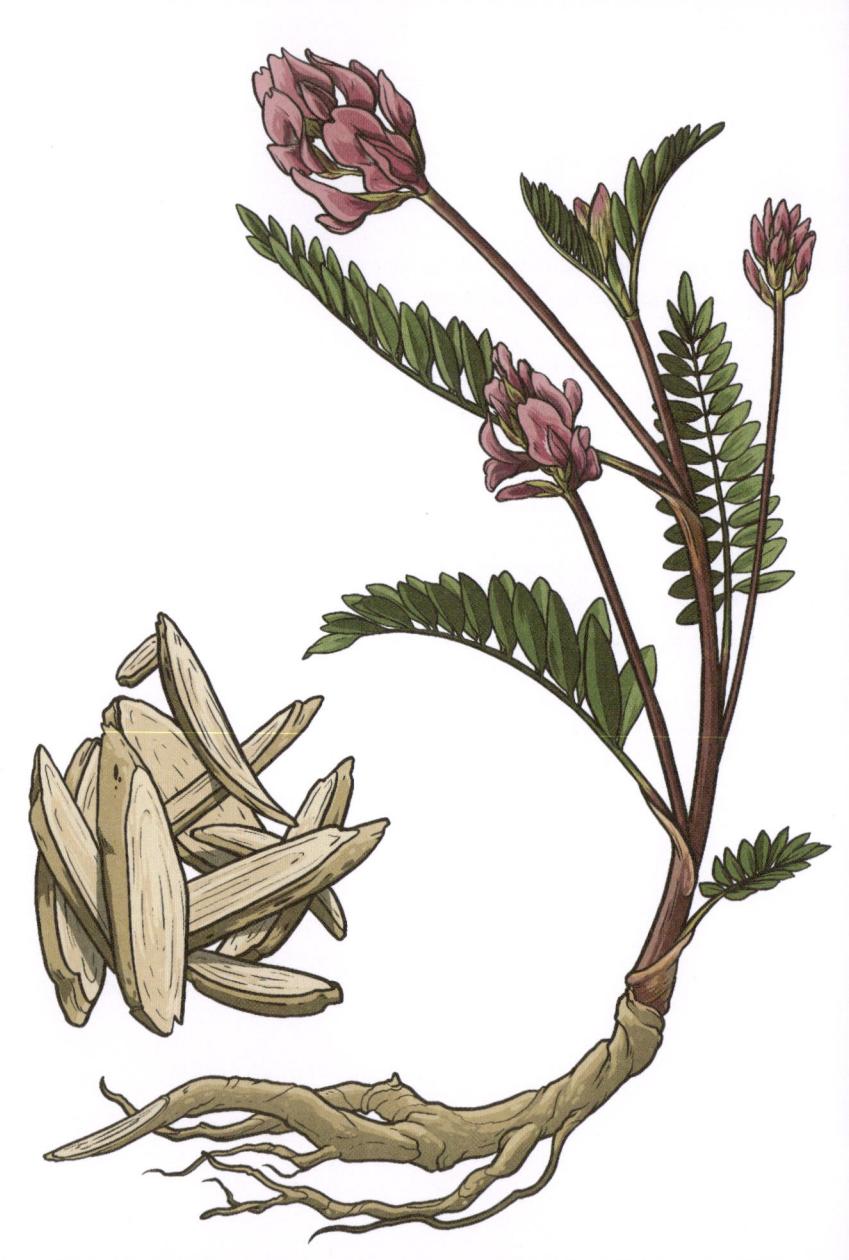

3

Astragalus

Astragalus membranaceus
Other name(s): *huang qi* (Chinese)

Astragalus holds great importance in Chinese medicine. In Traditional Chinese Medicine, every herb associates with specific organs. Astragalus corresponds to lungs and spleen, indicating its use for deficiencies in respiratory and digestive systems. This herb excels in supporting weak immune systems—those getting sick multiple times yearly with colds and flu. Take it between illnesses, not during. As an adaptogen, it builds immune resistance to stressors. The person who needs astragalus often experiences fatigue, loose stools, poor digestion, wheezing, edema, and frequent sweating. It uniquely helps nonhealing wounds such as sores and ulcers. Over time it can help with allergies in people with weakened immunity. It is best used as decoction or tincture.

PARTS USED: root

MEDICINAL USES: immunomodulation, adaptogenic, antiviral, anti-inflammatory, anti-tumor activity, diuretic

SAFETY CONSIDERATIONS: Avoid use during active colds or flu. This tonic remedy strengthens the system. When you are sick, use acute remedies instead to "kick the bug."

REMEDIES: Cold Kicking Vinegar, Immune Support Broth Blend, Stress Less Herbal Chai

TIP: Besides tea blends, add astragalus to broths, especially chicken broth! Common side effects from overuse or improper use include headaches, bloating, and dizziness (like inflating an already-full balloon). If these occur, reduce the dose or consider another herb.

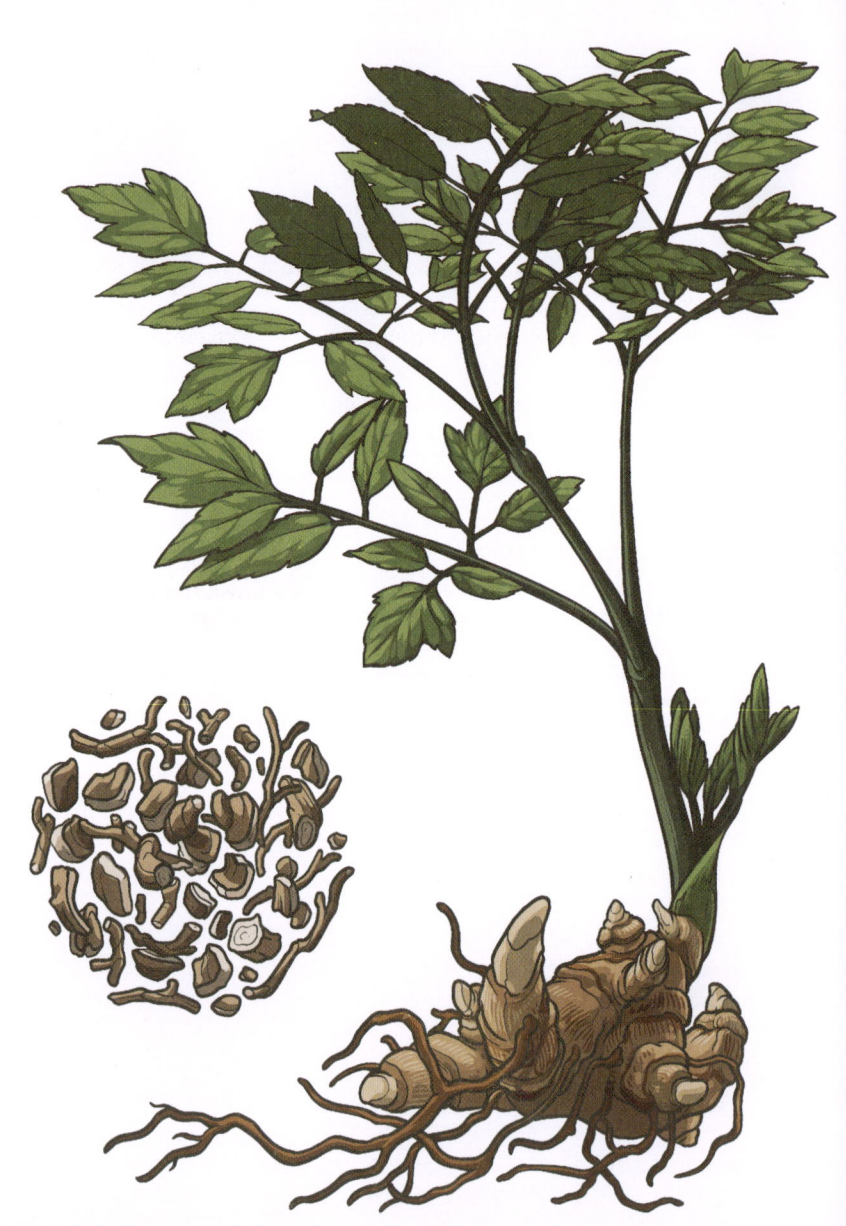

4

Black Cohosh

Cimicifuga racemosa or Actaea racemosa
Other name(s): bugbane, squawroot, snakeroot

Black cohosh has extensive Native American use for pregnancy and childbirth. The Algonquian word "cohosh" means "rough," possibly referring to the root's shape or rough leaves. This herb serves the female reproductive system throughout life—from menstruation through pregnancy to menopause. Clinical uses include menstrual cramps, pain, hormonal headaches, and menopausal complaints such as hot flashes. It also benefits the lungs, helping with painful coughs or lung dryness. It is best taken as a decoction, capsule, or tincture.

PARTS USED: root

MEDICINAL USES: antispasmodic, sedative, anti-inflammatory, analgesic, diuretic, estrogenic qualities

SAFETY CONSIDERATIONS: It is contraindicated during pregnancy, especially in the first trimester due to its emmena-gogue (promotes menstruation) effect. While rare clinically, reported side effects include slowed heart rate, nausea, vomiting, and other toxicity symptoms.

REMEDIES: Cramp Ease Elixir, Cool Me Down Hot Flash Tincture, Stop the Sweats Tincture

TIP: Start with lower doses to assess tolerance.

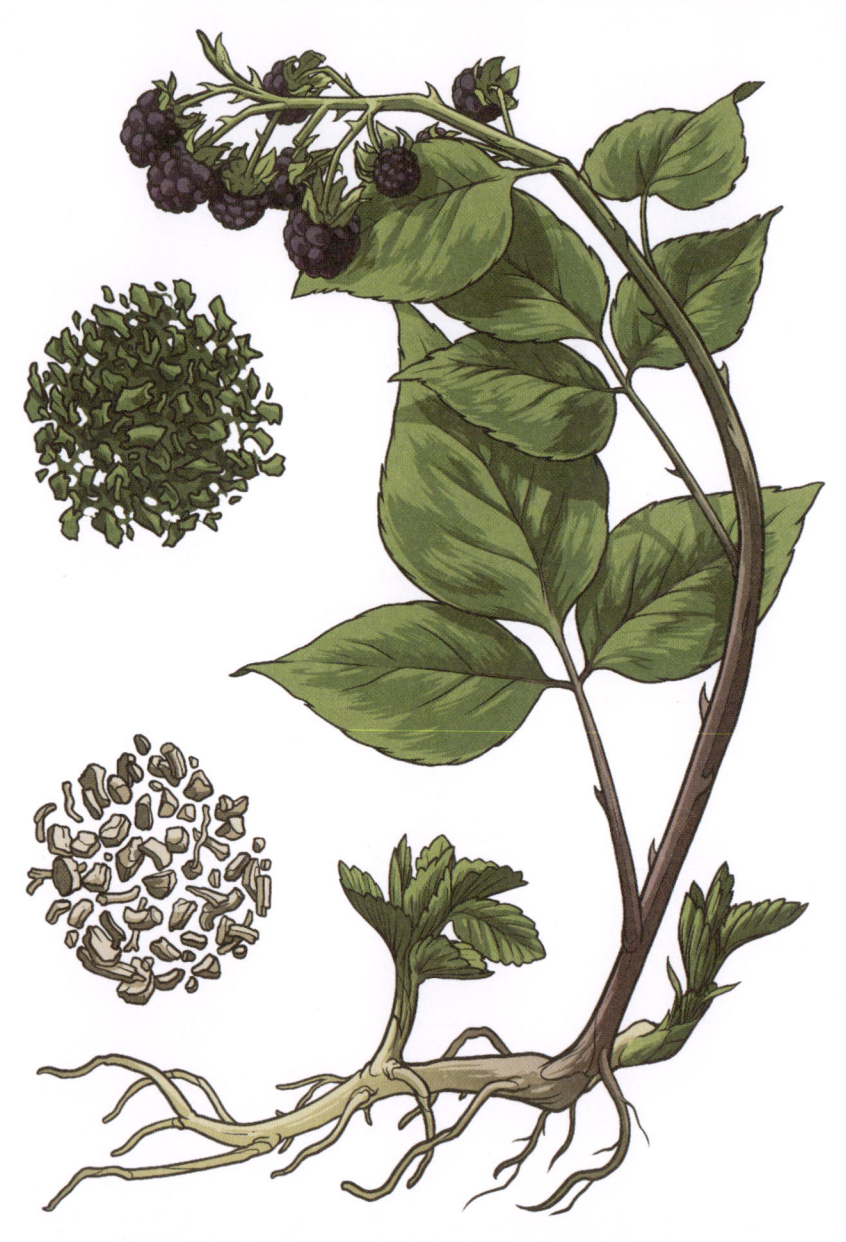

Blackberry

Rubus fruticosus, R. villosus
Other name(s): bramble, black brier

While most know blackberry for its delicious berries, this "pest" plant offers abundant medicine. The mineral-rich leaves provide astringent properties, treating conditions such as diarrhea or discharge—though root bark works more powerfully. Use leaf washes for minor skin conditions or use as a mouth/throat gargle for pain and inflammation. During pregnancy the leaves provide nourishment and support delivery. For leaves, take as infusions. For roots, take as a decoction or tincture.

PARTS USED: leaf and root (berries are edible)

MEDICINAL USES: astringent, anti-inflammatory, stops bleeding, nourishing, tonifies reproductive system

SAFETY CONSIDERATIONS: none noted

REMEDIES: Herbal Iron Syrup, Iron Tea, Plug It Up! Tincture, Rehydrating Tea for the Runs, Long Life Oxymel (optional addition), Sore Muscle Compress

TIP: Enjoy the whole plant! Eat the berries, dry the leaves, harvest the root, and scrape off the bark—it's a wonderful plant ally to know.

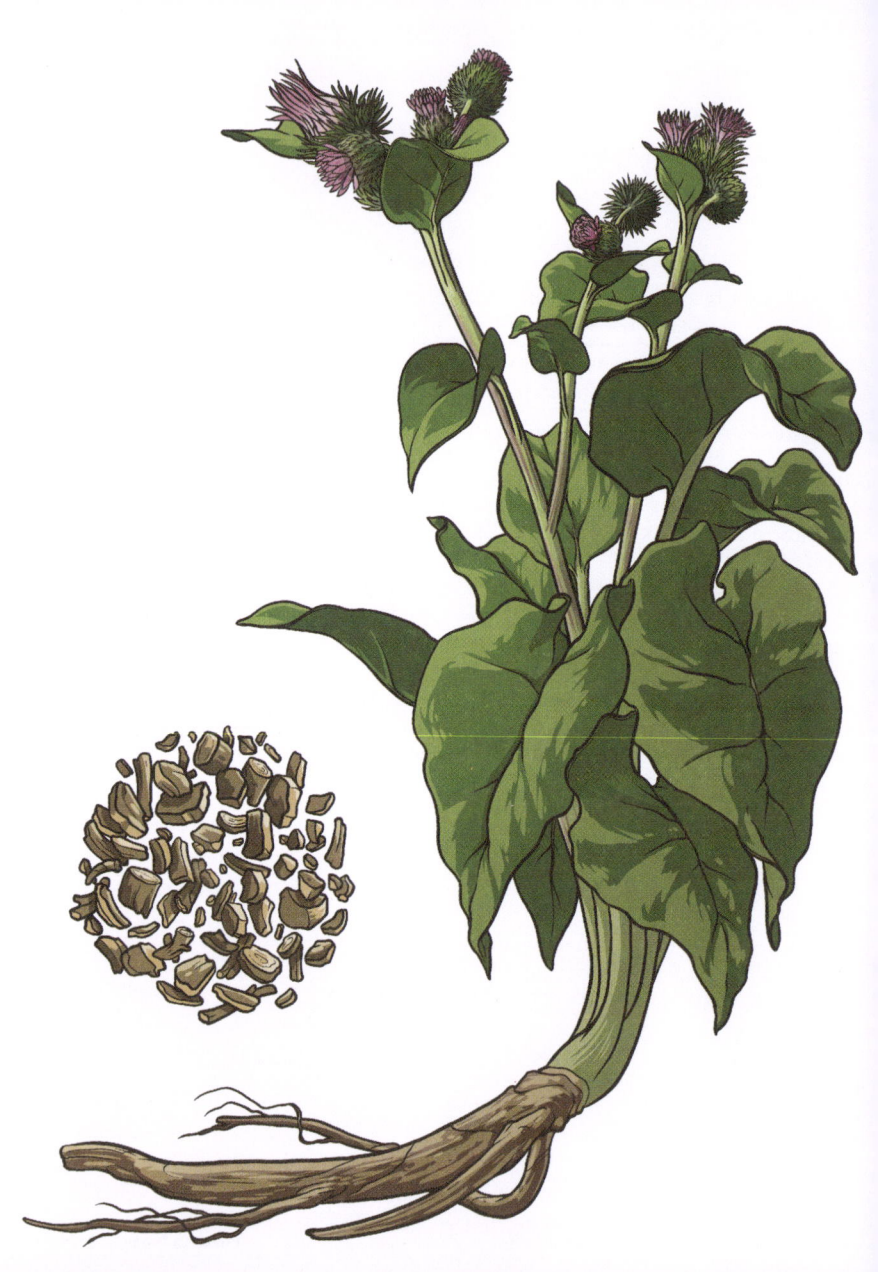

6

Burdock

Arctium lappa
Other name(s): *Gobo* (Japanese)

Burdock has many uses. This sweet yet bitter, slightly mucilaginous plant looks like a thin, white, hairy carrot in your grocery store. But try it in a stir-fry! The dried root is excellent for skin, lymph, digestion, and liver support. Many bitter formulas include burdock to stimulate digestion, and it helps balance blood sugar. The root's high inulin content benefits gut flora. It also contains polysaccharides, tannins, and minerals like calcium, phosphorus, sodium, and iron. It is best taken as a decoction, tincture, or food.

PARTS USED: root

MEDICINAL USES: anti-inflammatory, antibacterial, antifungal, diuretic, digestive stimulant, lymphatic circulation, mild laxative

SAFETY CONSIDERATIONS: Use with caution during pregnancy due to its oxytocic effects.

REMEDIES: Gentle Liver Tonic Tea for Acne, Cholesterol Helper Tea, Blood Sugar Stabilizer Tea, Shiny Happy Hair Tea, Flaky Scalp Hair Rinse, Women's Rooted Tea, Digestive Bitters, Gentle Liver Detox Formula, Psoriasis Relief Tea, Root Beer Syrup

TIP: A tea made with equal parts burdock, rose petals, and nettles is a wonderful daily blend—give it a try!

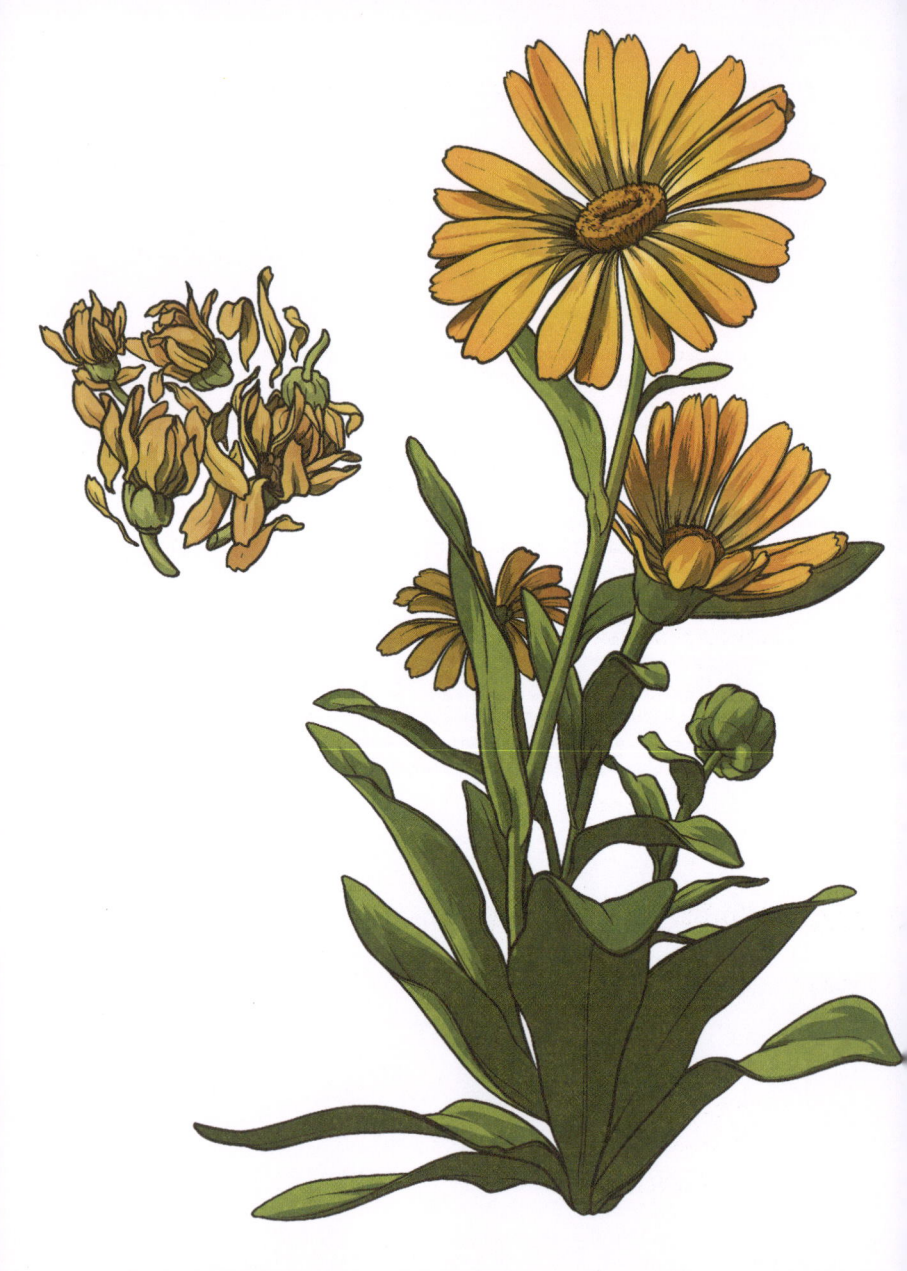

7

Calendula

Calendula officinalis

Other name(s): It is sometimes called "marigold" in literature—
use caution, as most marigolds are ornamental, inedible, and
highly toxic!

Calendula provides abundant healing. The flower tastes slightly
bitter, salty, and drying, yet remains lovely and mild in tea. Most
popular for skin conditions due to its anti-inflammatory, antiseptic,
and antibacterial properties. Gentle enough for babies and children.
Use in washes, baths, and oils externally. Internally it addresses
lymphatic congestion—excellent for skin issues such as acne
related to lymph and liver. It is best used as tea (internal or external), tincture, or succus (juiced plant).

PARTS USED: flower

MEDICINAL USES: antiseptic,
anti-inflammatory, lymphagogue,
wound-healing, antibacterial,
liver tonic

SAFETY CONSIDERATIONS: Use
with caution during pregnancy
due to its possible emmenagogue effects. Always clean
wounds before applying to
prevent trapping bacteria.

REMEDIES: Reflux Relief Tea,
Gentle Liver Tonic Tea for Acne,
Acne Healing Vinegar, Dry
Those Drips Tea, Sore Bum Sitz
Bath (alternative option), Kick
That Cold Sore Tea, Cooling
Calendula Eye Compress, Herbal
Foot Soak for Tired Feet, Hemmy
Soothe Herbal Wash, Immune
Support Broth Blend, Fertili-Tea,
Lymph Mover Tea, Postpartum
Sitz Bath, After Birth Rebalance
Tea, Calendula Wash for Irritated
Skin, Beautiful Skin Herbal Facial
Steam, Floral Herbal Toner,
Calendula Comfrey Skin Salve,
Soothing Spirit Herbal Bath,
Flaky Scalp Hair Rinse, Gentle
Eczema Helper Tea, Herbal Bath
for Itchy Skin

TIP: Harvest flowers when
fully open on sunny days for
maximum potency.

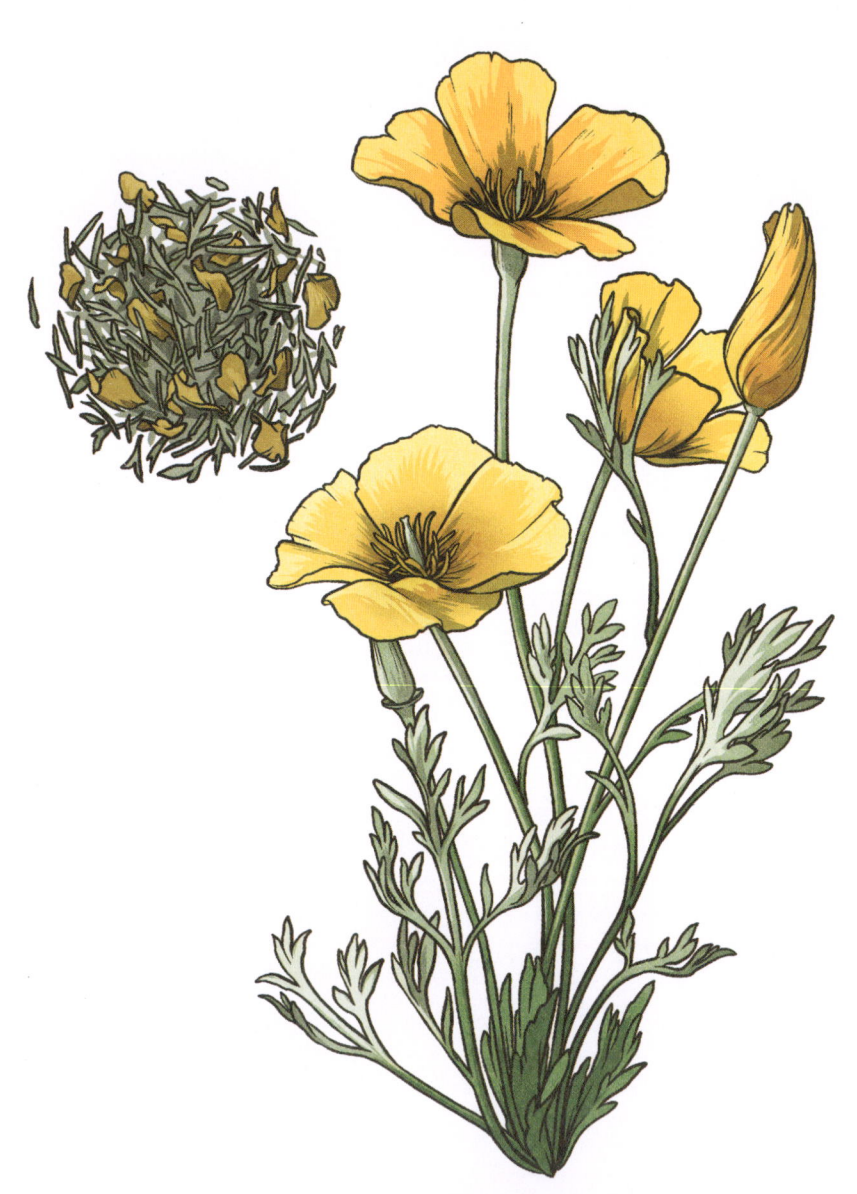

8

California Poppy

Eschscholzia californica
Other name(s): none commonly used

These bright orange flowers bring joy every summer when scattered along highways (though roadside plants aren't ideal for harvesting due to pollution). This plant wasn't a regular in the repertoire until working with pain patients revealed its excellence. Bitter and cooling, with an affinity for heart and liver, it excels in treating pain, especially neck and upper back. It is also helpful for stress, anxiety, insomnia, and spasmodic conditions such as coughing. It is very calming for the mind—Native Americans historically used it for children with colic, insomnia, and restlessness. It is best used as an infusion or tincture.

PARTS USED: aerial parts (also root, but above-ground is most important)

MEDICINAL USES: sedative, analgesic, antispasmodic

SAFETY CONSIDERATIONS: Use it cautiously during pregnancy due to its uterine-stimulating effects from the alkaloid, cryptopine.

REMEDIES: Passionflower Tincture for Anxiety (optional addition), Get to Sleep Tea, Pain Relieving Tea

TIP: Unlike its opium poppy cousin, California poppy is gentle and nonaddictive.

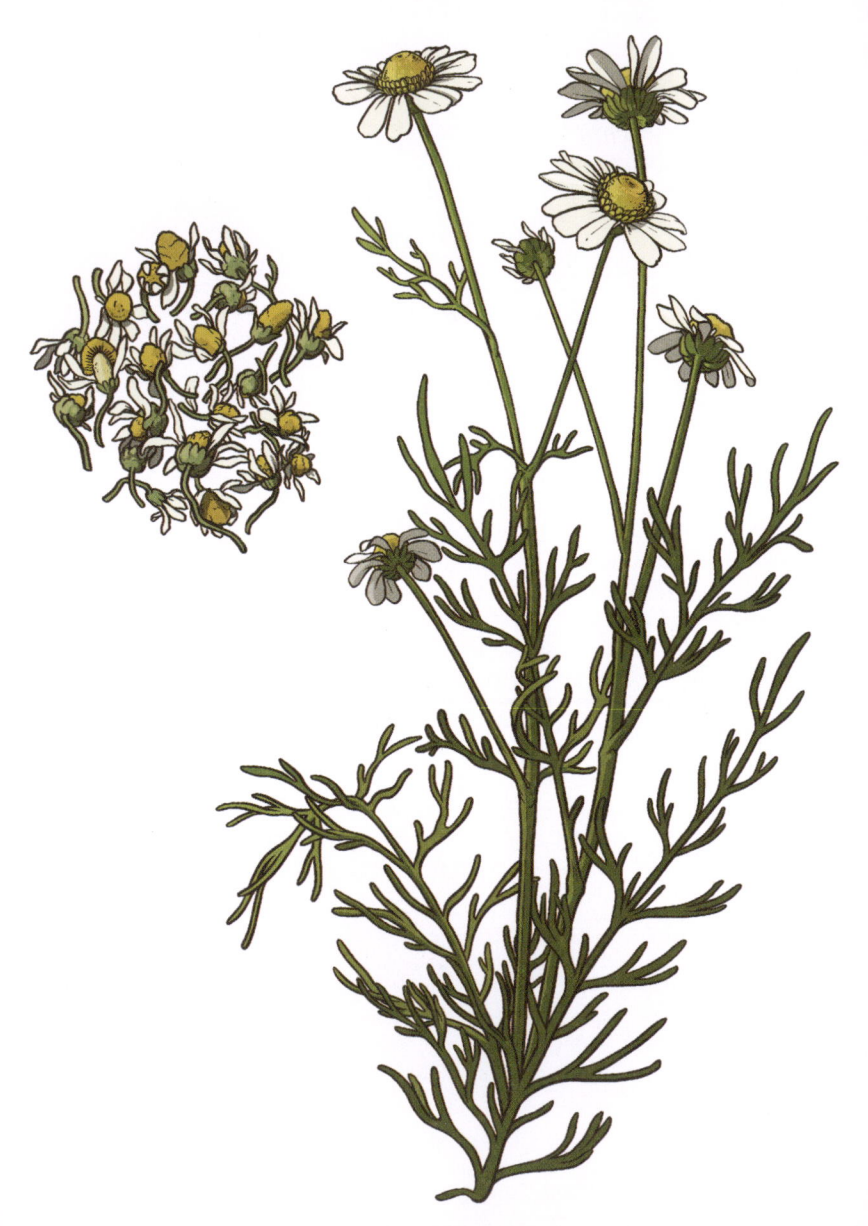

Chamomile

Matricaria recutita and Anthemis nobilis

Other name(s): German chamomile (*Matricaria recutita*), Roman chamomile (*Anthemis nobilis*)

Chamomile quickly became a favorite when herbalism studies began. Moving beyond bagged tea (just herb dust!) to real dried chamomile buds reveals a taste like eating a honeyed cookie while lying in the sun—warm, sweet, and healing. Perfect for anxious, nervous, irritable, or restless people (like uncomfortable babies needing comfort from warm chamomile tea!). As an antispasmodic, it helps tight, spasmed muscles and pain. Excellent for digestion, soothing upset stomach, nausea, or gas. Use topically as a wash as you would use calendula. It is best used as an infusion or tincture.

PARTS USED: flowers

MEDICINAL USES: antispasmodic, anti-inflammatory, analgesic, antifungal, sedative, carminative, wound healing

SAFETY CONSIDERATIONS: Some people may have allergic sensitivity, though this is rarely seen clinically.

REMEDIES: Reflux Relief Tea, Acne Healing Vinegar, Anxie-Tea, Cramp Ease Tea, Cramp Ease Elixir, Easy Mover Tea (Constipation), Tummy Ease Tea, Soothing Tummy Gummies, Goodbye Gas Tea, Headache Relief Tea, Hemmy Soothe Herbal Wash, Digestive Bitters, Jaw Clench Relief Poultice, Pain Relieving Tea, Herbal Bath for Itchy Skin, Herbal Skin Oil for Dry Skin, Stress Relief Tea, Floral Herbal Toner, Sore Muscle Compress (optional addition), Soothing Spirit Herbal Bath

TIP: Wild feverfew resembles wild chamomile. Both look like tiny white daisies, but chamomile has delicate, wispy leaves.

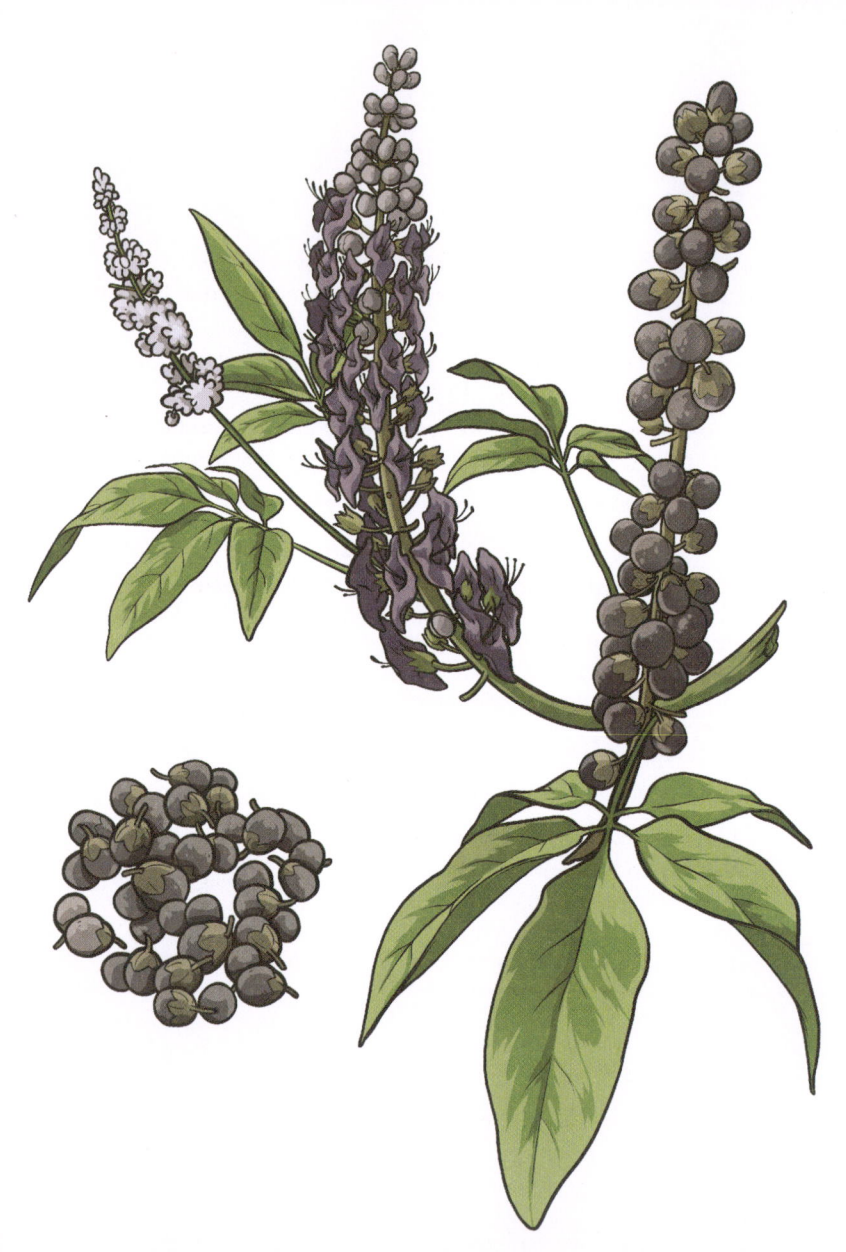

10

Chaste Tree Berry

Vitex agnus castus
Other name(s): vitex, monk's pepper, cloister pepper

Chaste tree berry has long addressed hormonal ailments. According to Dr. Sharol Tilgner, this herb increases luteinizing hormone (peaking around ovulation) and inhibits follicle-stimulating hormone release. It helps with PMS, cramping, hormonal acne, and menopausal symptoms. It is also very helpful for stabilizing hormones when discontinuing birth control. I find it useful for those who are coming off birth control to stabilize their hormones. It has a spicy, peppercorn-like taste and is best used as a long infusion or a tincture.

PARTS USED: dried fruit (berry)

MEDICINAL USES: harmonizes and regulates the menstrual cycle, helps with menopausal symptoms, helpful with progesterone deficiencies, antispasmodic, warming, drying

SAFETY CONSIDERATIONS: It is contraindicated for use during pregnancy due to it emmenagogue effect. It may counteract effectiveness of birth control pills and some hormone therapy.

REMEDIES: Women's Rooted Tea, After Birth Rebalance Tea

TIP: While chaste tree berry appears in a few tea formulas in this book, it can also be taken on its own in tincture form. A standard dose is two dropperfuls, twice daily, for up to three menstrual cycles. Monitor for any changes during that time.

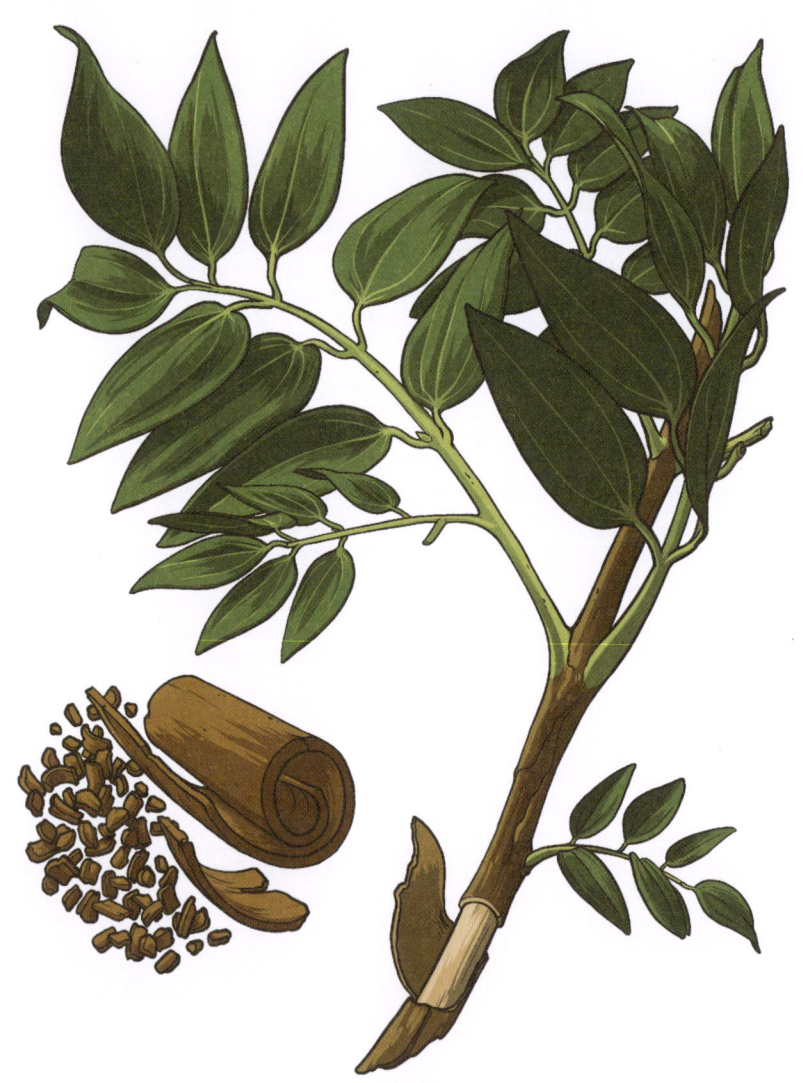

11

Cinnamon

Cinnamomum spp.

Other name(s): cassia chips, *gui zhi* (twig parts in Chinese),
rou gui (bark in Chinese)

Cinnamon is a common household herb—spicy, aromatic, sweet,
drying, and stimulating. In Chinese herbal medicine, various parts
(twigs or bark) serve different medicinal purposes. Whether using
Ceylon cinnamon sticks or cassia chips, expect similar warming,
pain-relieving, blood sugar stabilizing, and aromatic qualities. If
you use it as a kitchen herb for flavoring, you're already receiving
medicinal benefits! It is best used as a long infusion, decoction,
or tincture.

PARTS USED: bark and twigs

MEDICINAL USES: warming,
astringing, carminative, antibacterial, antifungal, pain-relieving,
blood sugar stabilizing

SAFETY CONSIDERATIONS:
Be careful using large doses
over long periods of time. Use
essential oil with caution, as it
may cause burning (never apply
directly to the skin or in baths).

REMEDIES: Blood Sugar Stabilizer
Tea, Cough Syrup, Dry Cough
Tea, Cold Kicker Tea, Warm Me
Up Tea, Women's Rooted Tea,
Healing Heart Syrup, Dreamer's
Cordial, Stress Less Herbal Chai

TIP: For tea blends, cassia
chips work better than whole
cinnamon sticks, which don't
steep well.

NOTE: "Spp" at the end of this
latin taxonomy means "species."
Latin names here are shown as
"Genus, Species," and when
a plant has multiple species,
we write "spp" at the end to
indicate this.

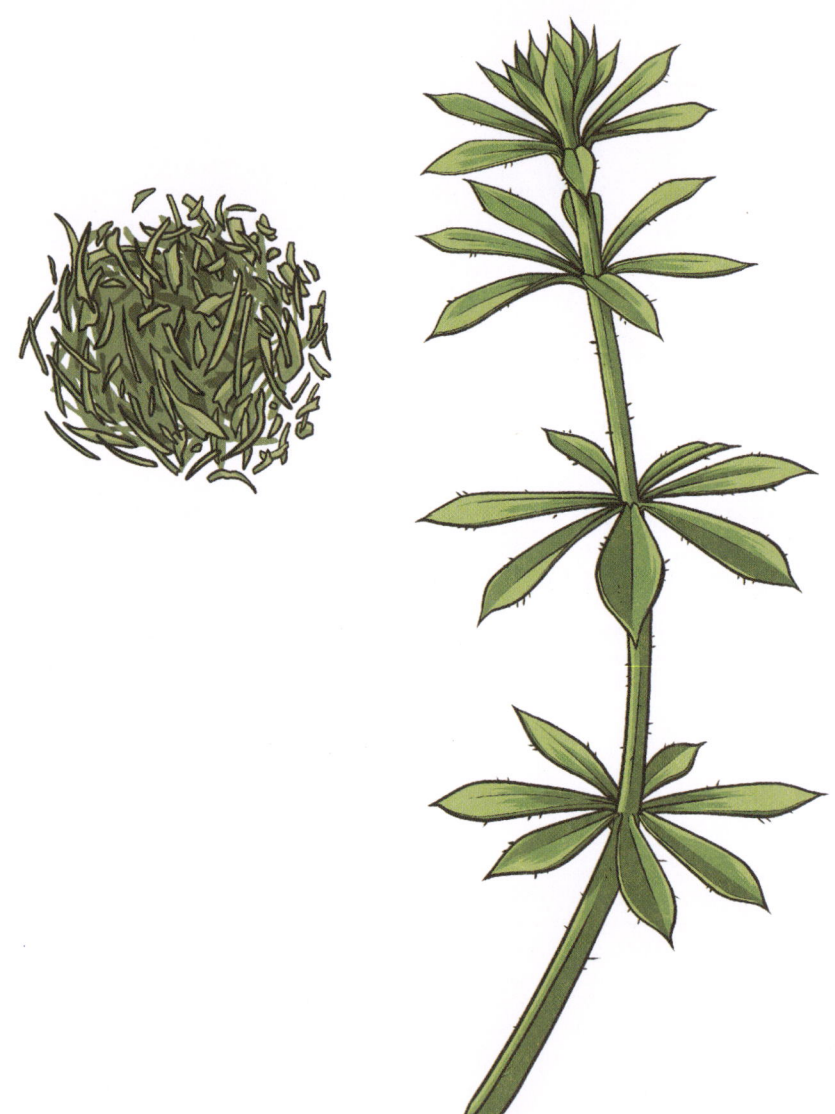

Cleavers

Galium aparine

Other name(s): goosegrass, catchweed, stickyweed, cleaverwort

Walkers and hikers know cleavers—or rather, cleavers know them, sticking to pants like Velcro! Bright green, long, and spindly with sticky leaves, this cooling and drying plant helps stagnant lymphatic systems, clears skin, harmonizes urinary symptoms, and supports detoxification. Some find it helpful for toxic heat conditions such as abscesses, sores, or bacterial infections (though not as a sole treatment). Fresh juice works best, but dried tea remains helpful. Cleavers are best prepared as fresh juice, infusions, or tinctures.

PARTS USED: aerial parts

MEDICINAL USES: diuretic, nutritive, lymphagogue, anti-inflammatory, wound healing

SAFETY CONSIDERATIONS: none noted

REMEDIES: Lymph Mover Tea, Psoriasis Relief Tea

TIP: Harvest cleavers in spring when they are young and tender for juicing—older plants become tough and less effective.

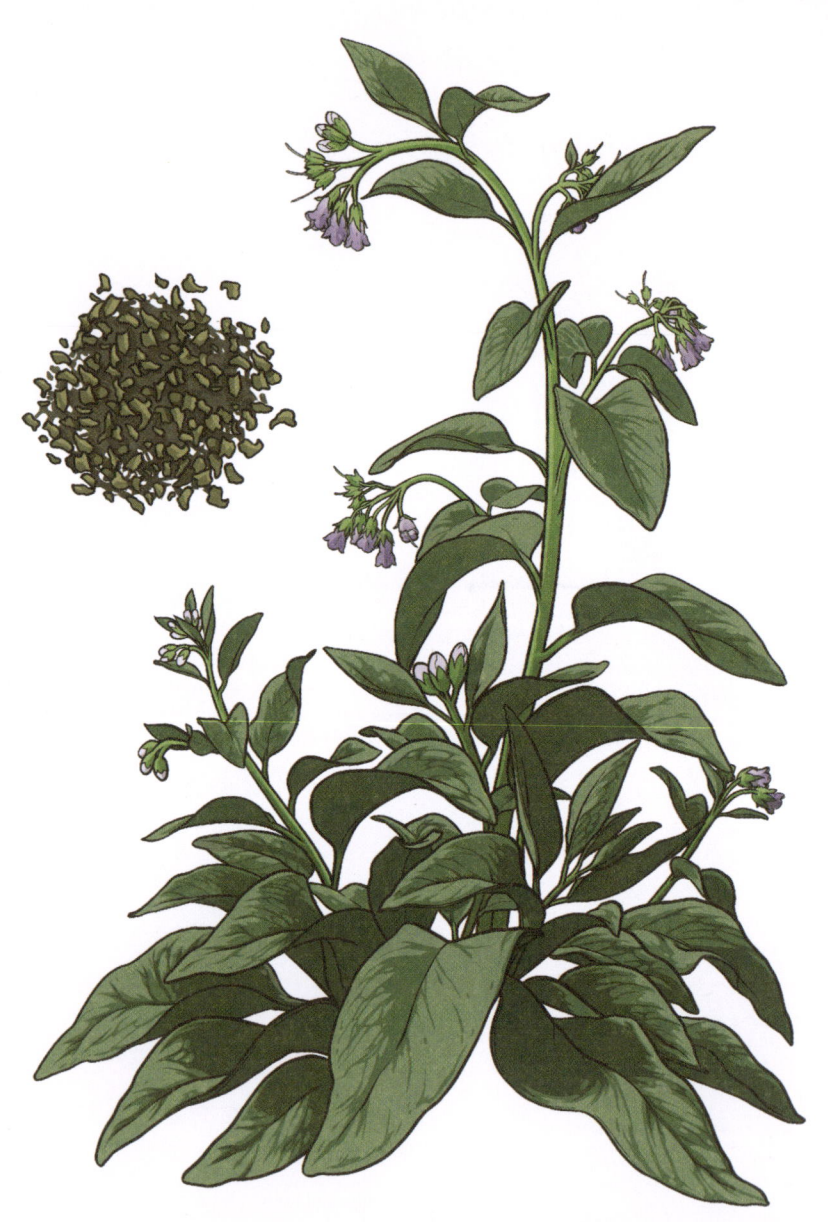

Comfrey

Symphytum officinalis
Other name(s): knitbone

Comfrey initially inspired caution! Despite its long history as an incredible wound healer, the compound pyrrolizidine alkaloids (toxic to liver) placed it on many contraindication lists. Understanding both its dangers and benefits allows responsible use. It is high in vitamins A and C, silicon, selenium, potassium, riboflavin, and more. Use externally as poultice for bone healing, fractures, and skin ulcerations (hence "knitbone"). It is best used fresh or dried for poultices.

PARTS USED: leaf and root

MEDICINAL USES: mucilaginous, wound healing, astringent, anti-inflammatory, demulcent

SAFETY CONSIDERATIONS: Use with caution internally due to the pyrrolizidine and its toxicity warnings.

REMEDIES: Mugwort Healing Liniment, Hemmy Soothe Herbal Wash (optional addition), Herbal Foot Soak, Postpartum Sitz Bath, Floral Herbal Toner, Calendula Comfrey Skin Salve, Sore Muscle Compress

TIP: Try making this as a stand-alone herbal oil—it transforms into a beautiful, vibrant green.

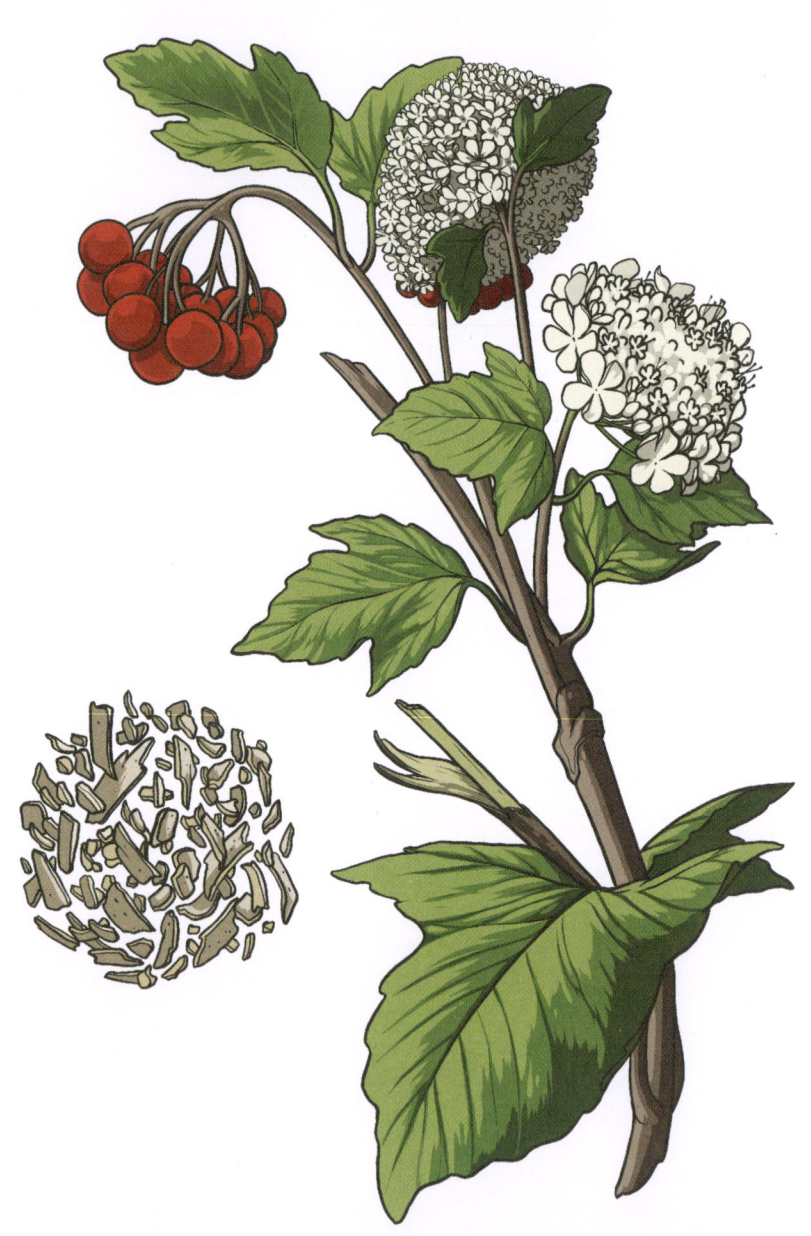

Cramp Bark

Viburnum opulus or V. prunifolium
Other name(s): guelder rose, snowball tree

As the name suggests, cramp bark excels for cramps! The bark is astringent, aromatic, and drying. When flowering, blossoms resemble snowballs—beautiful white blooms similar to hydrangeas. The bark commonly treats menstrual cramping but works for any spasmodic cramping and pain. Its astringent quality helps when pelvic cramps accompany heavy blood loss. It is best used as a long infusion, decoction, or tincture. Having a tincture handy allows taking 1 to 2 dropperfuls every 15 to 30 minutes for cramping relief.

PARTS USED: bark

MEDICINAL USES: antispasmodic, astringent, nervous system relaxant, carminative, anti-inflammatory

SAFETY CONSIDERATIONS: Avoid using with blood thinning medications due to the coumarin constituents of the plant. Use cautiously during pregnancy (unless under the care of a knowledgeable provider, as it is occasionally helpful in labor prep). The berries are extremely toxic.

REMEDIES: Cramp Ease Tea, Cramp Ease Elixir

TIP: Harvest bark in spring or fall when the plant energy concentrates there, not during active growth.

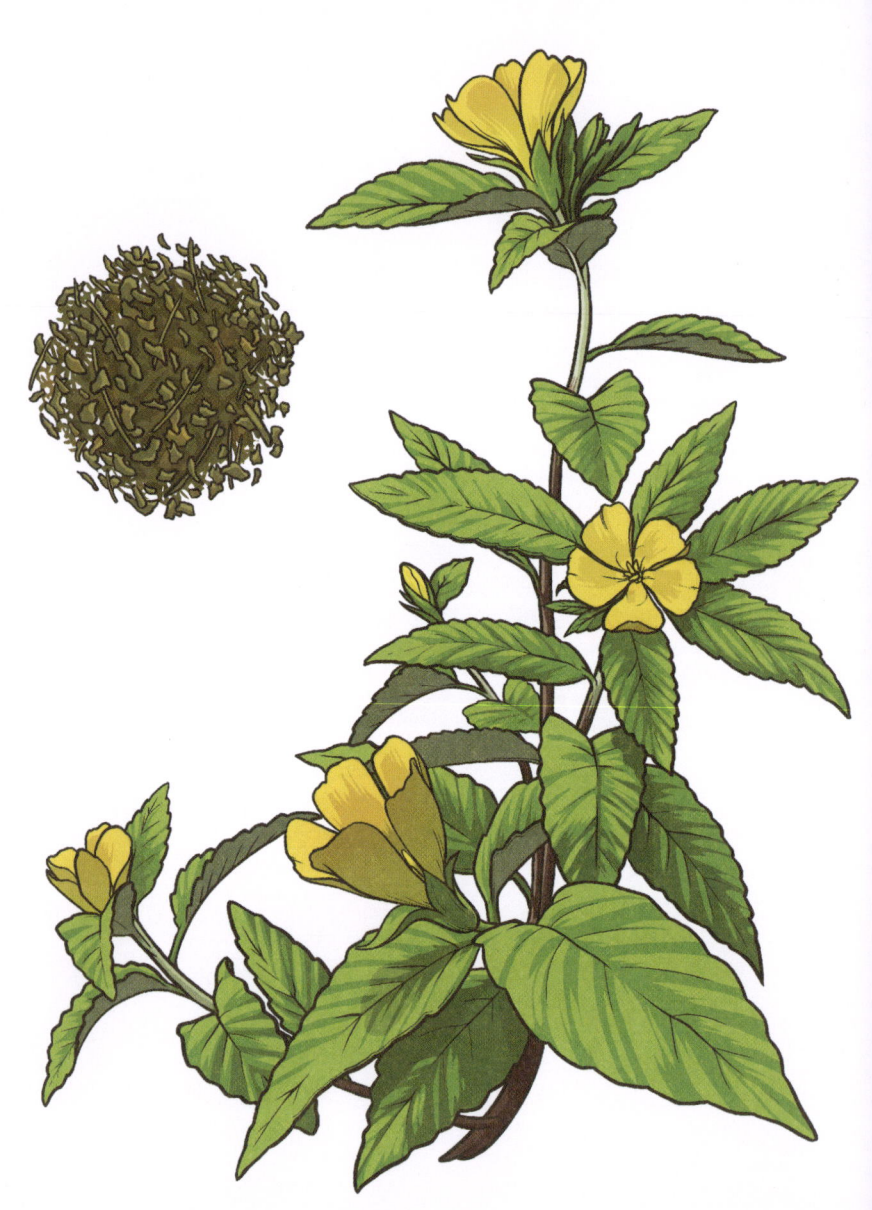

Damiana

Turnera diffusa
Other name(s): none commonly used

Damiana is known for its aphrodisiac abilities and its slightly bitter, herbaceous, almost resinous taste. It is most useful as a warming and uplifting aphrodisiac that tonifies reproductive organs. Proven helpful as an antidepressant, it lifts mood and addresses chronic depression and fatigue. As an expectorant, it helps colds and coughs with excess mucus. Mark Pedersen's *Nutritional Herbology* notes its incredible nutrients—highest in chromium and zinc, followed by vitamins A and C—and calls it a blood purifier. It is best used as tea or tincture.

PARTS USED: aerial parts

MEDICINAL USES: aphrodisiac, nutritive, nervous system stimulant, blood purifier, expectorant

SAFETY CONSIDERATIONS: Use with caution during pregnancy due to its stimulating effects.

REMEDIES: Uplifting Nervous System Tonic, In-the-Mood Damiana Cordial, Dreamer's Cordial, Let the Sun In Tea

TIP: Try this herb on its own as a tincture. Just a few drops in the morning can help lift the mood and provide a gentle sense of warmth—especially on cold, damp winter days!

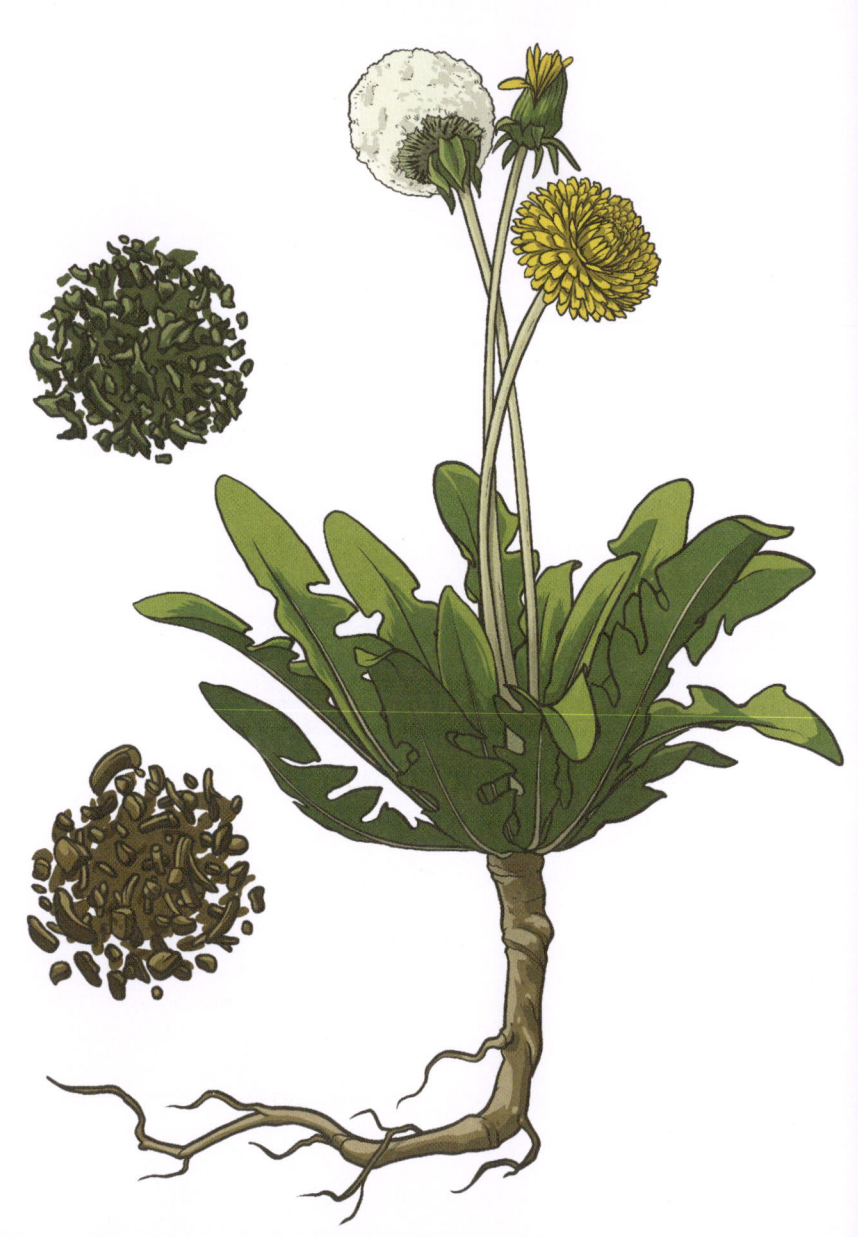

Dandelion

Taraxacum officinalis
Other name(s): puffball, lion's tooth

Nature's way of saying everyone needs this plant—the dandelion grows as a "weed" everywhere! The whole plant serves medicinally, though its leaves and roots predominate. Roasted root can make a warming coffee substitute. Dandelion wine, an old folk recipe, ferments blossoms with sugar, sometimes citrus or raisins, creating a mild, tasty beverage. Leaves and roots provide diuretic action, support skin health, and aid digestion. The root contains inulin, a beneficial gut bacteria. It is rich in potassium, iron, manganese, sodium, vitamin A, and many other nutrients. This potassium content is especially helpful for conditions needing diuretic support such as edema or hypertension. The leaf is best used as an infusion. The root is best used as a long infusion or decoction. Tinctures work well too.

PARTS USED: leaves and root (some folk remedies will use the blossoms)

MEDICINAL USES: diuretic, mild laxative, helpful for the liver, helpful for cholesterol, blood purifier

SAFETY CONSIDERATIONS: Contact with the fresh plant may cause dermatitis in some individuals.

REMEDIES: Lymph Mover Tea, Gentle Liver Detox Formula, Digestive Bitters, Immune Support Broth Blend, Women's Rooted Tea, Long Life Oxymel, Root Beer Syrup, Daily Multivitamin Tea, Cholesterol Helper Tea, Blood Sugar Stabilizer Tea, Bye-Bye Bloat Tea, Arthritis Alleviation Tea, Iron Tea, Herbal Iron Syrup, Gentle Liver Tonic Tea for Acne

TIP: Look for dandelion in grocery products such as coffee substitutes, kombucha, or low-sugar sodas—herbal medicine hiding in plain sight!

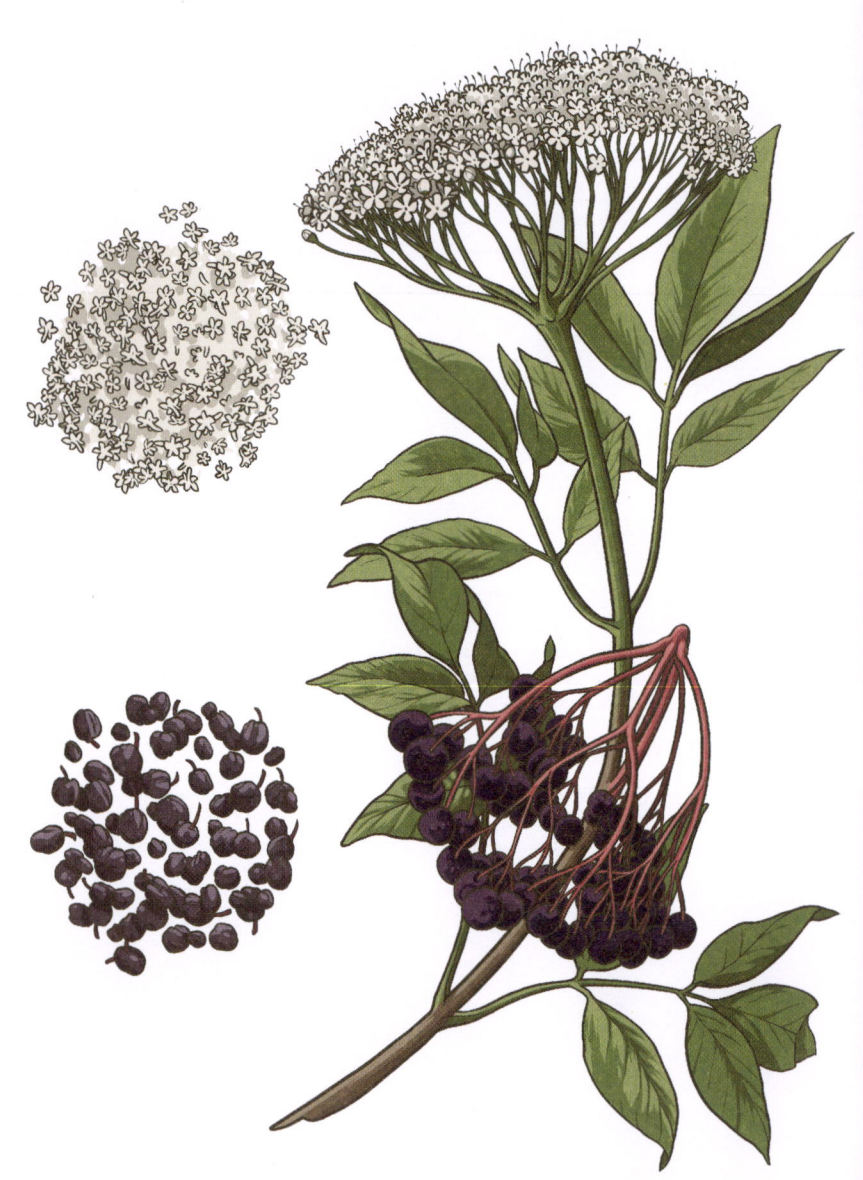

Elder

Sambucus nigra
Other name(s): black elder, pipe tree, bore tree, bour tree

Natural grocery stores showcase elderberry syrup and *Sambucus* products. These berries and flowers offer immune support and much more! Berries stimulate immunity and help with coughs and mucus. The tiny, fairylike star flowers work as diaphoretics—helping vent early-stage fevers. This "up and out" action also helps with headaches and allergies. Corinne Boyer's *Under the Witching Tree* notes that "the whole tree was considered a supernatural nature spirit since ancient times" with a long magical practice history. *Sambucus nigra*, black elderberry, predominates in herbal medicine. Berries are best used as decoction, long infusion, or syrup. Flowers are best used as an infusion.

PARTS USED: flower, berry

MEDICINAL USES: immune stimulant, diaphoretic (flowers), diuretic, expectorant, mild laxative (berries)

SAFETY CONSIDERATIONS: none noted for proper preparations

REMEDIES: Dry Those Drips Tea, Cold Kicker Tea, Fever Diminish Tea, Floral Herbal Toner

TIP: Elderberry syrup is simple to make—follow the syrup recipe guide and use just elderberries! Add cinnamon stick, star anise, hawthorn berry, and rose hips for variety.

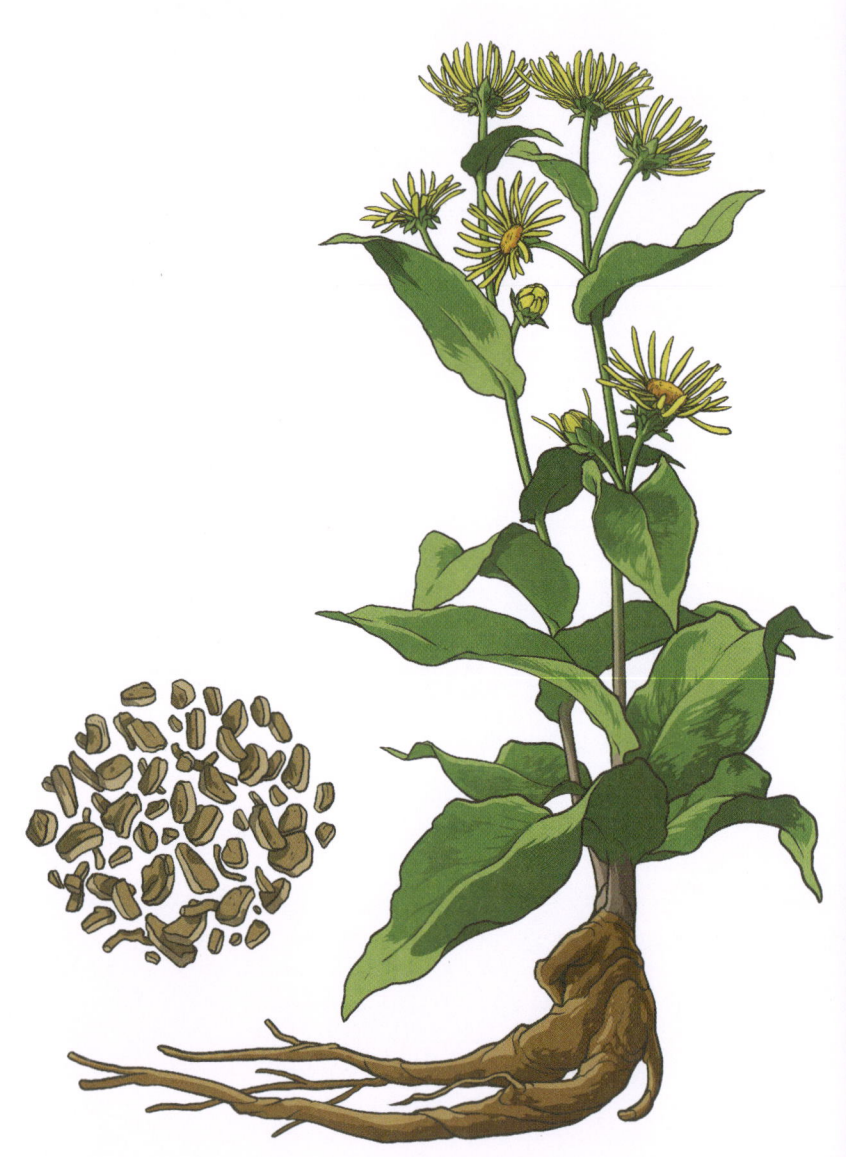

Elecampane

Inula helenium
Other name(s): elfwort, elfdock, horseheal

Elecampane stands tall with bright yellow flowers. The root—aromatic, pungent, sweet, slightly warming, drying, and stimulating—features in historical wine recipes and candied preparations for respiratory, throat, and stomach conditions. It is clinically useful for chronic, phlegmy coughs in tea or syrup form. It can slowly tonify lungs and stomach over time. It can be helpful for immune depletion with fatigue. Though less commonly used this way, it reportedly "promotes menstruation and increases hormones," helping with PMS symptoms such as tender breasts, dry skin, and irritability. Elecampane can brighten spirits after a long illness. It is best used as a decoction, syrup, or tincture.

PARTS USED: root

MEDICINAL USES: antiseptic, expectorant, carminative, diaphoretic, immunostimulant, anti-inflammatory, helpful for the digestive system

SAFETY CONSIDERATIONS: Avoid large doses, which may cause vomiting and diarrhea. Avoid use during pregnancy as it is a uterine stimulant.

REMEDIES: Cough Syrup, Dry Cough Tea (optional addition)

TIP: If you're ever able to get the fresh root, try making an elixir with alcohol and honey! It's both delicious and soothing to the spirit. (Dried root can work as well, though fresh is preferred.)

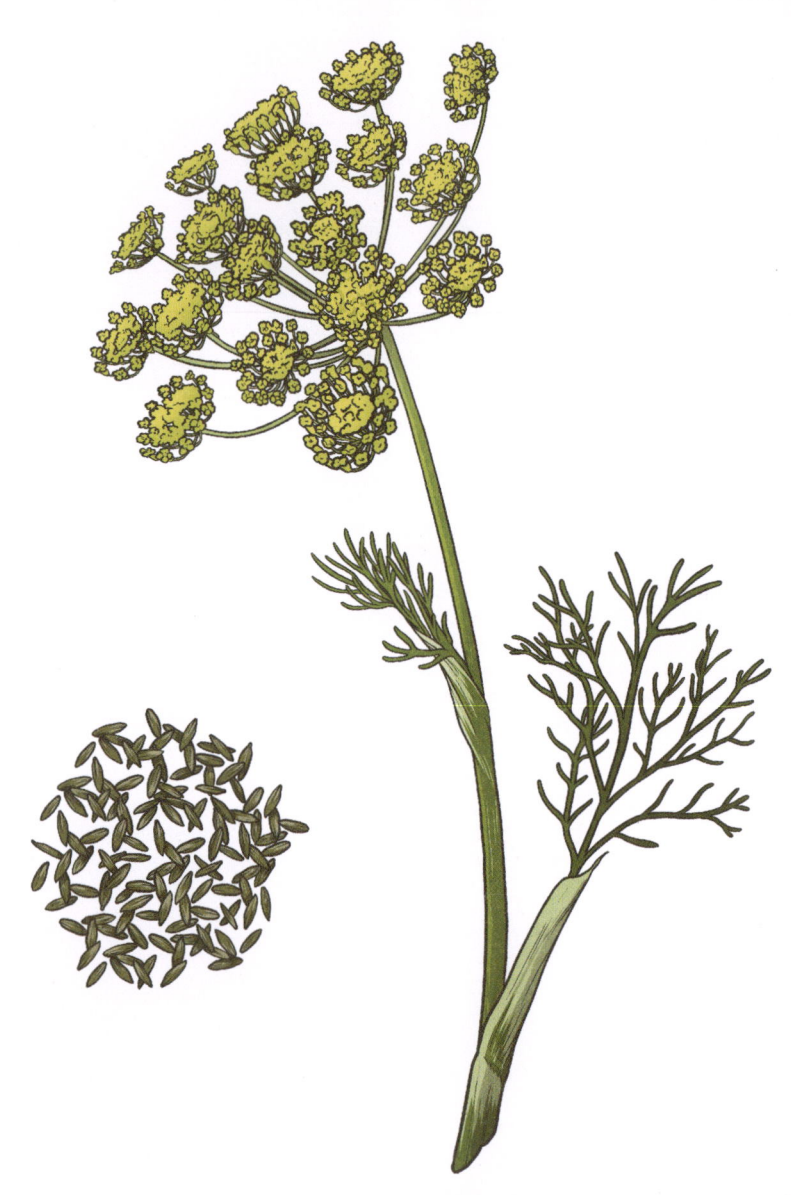

Fennel

Foeniculum vulgare
Other name(s): sweet fennel, wild fennel

Fennel belongs to the carrot family, and tends to be a tall, stalky plant with beautiful flower clusters called umbels (like inside-out umbrellas!). The aromatic, sweet, spicy, warming seeds excel for digestive complaints such as gas and indigestion, even mildly suppressing appetite. Its light expectorant action helps clear mucus during coughs and colds. Medieval times saw fennel and St. John's wort hung over doors to prevent witchcraft and evil influences. Many cultures embrace this herb: Chinese medicine uses it similarly, Indian restaurants offer candied seeds after meals for digestion, Italian cooking features it prominently (remember fennel biscotti at the holidays?). The taste delights! It is best used as an infusion.

PARTS USED: seeds

MEDICINAL USES: carminative, antispasmodic, diuretic, expectorant

SAFETY CONSIDERATIONS: It is contraindicated during pregnancy due to its emmenagogue effect.

REMEDIES: Reflux Relief Tea, Easy Mover Tea, Cough Syrup, Dry Cough Tea, Tummy Ease Tea, Happy Lungs Tea, Herbal Bath for Itchy Skin, Goodbye Gas Tea, Stress Less Herbal Chai

TIP: Try adding fennel to your tea blends for a little sweetness. Explore recipes such as fennel biscotti—and incorporate more herbs into your daily cooking!

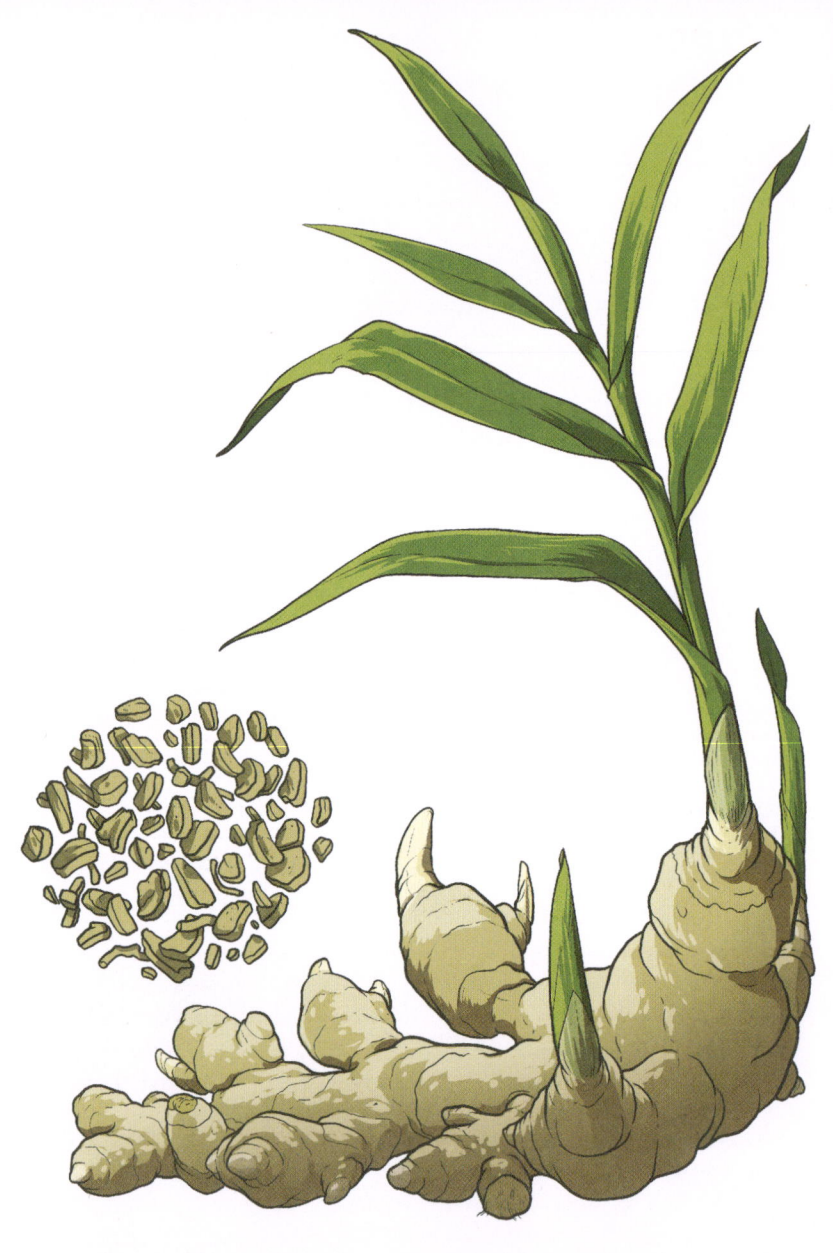

Ginger

Zingiber officinalis
Other name(s): *Sheng jiang* (the fresh root in Chinese),
gan jiang (the dried root in Chinese)

This spicy, warming herb proves invaluable when kept handy.
Beneficial for the digestive system, it also helps with arthritis, pain,
circulation, motion sickness, first trimester nausea, and inflammation. Remember using ginger ale for upset stomachs? Now you know
why! Gentle enough for daily use by all ages. The Chinese add it to
food and sip fresh ginger tea at meals. It is best used fresh or dried
for decoction or long infusion.

PARTS USED: root

MEDICINAL USES: anti-
inflammatory, carminative,
diaphoretic, diuretic, antispasmodic, antioxidant, analgesic,
expectorant

SAFETY CONSIDERATIONS:
Large doses are contraindicated
during pregnancy.

REMEDIES: Arthritis Alleviation
Tea, Ginger Soak for Arthritic
Hands, Digestive Bitters,
Women's Rooted Tea, Warm Me
Up Tea, Root Beer Syrup, Cold
Kicking Vinegar, Cholesterol
Helper Tea, Blood Sugar
Stabilizer Tea, Cold Kicker Tea,
Easy Mover Tea, Cough Syrup,
Tummy Ease Tea, Goodbye
Gas Tea, Healing Heart Syrup,
Hangover Hydration Tea,
Soothing Tea for Nausea
Pain Relieving Tea, Ginger Tea for
Nausea, After Birth Rebalance
Tea, Stress Less Herbal Chai,
Cramp Ease Tea

TIP: Try experimenting with
different ways to prepare ginger.
One method is to use the edge
of a spoon to gently scrape off
the skin. You can also slice it
into dime-sized rounds or grate
it using the fine side of a grater,
which helps release some of its
juice. Choose the method that
works best for your recipes and
cooking style!

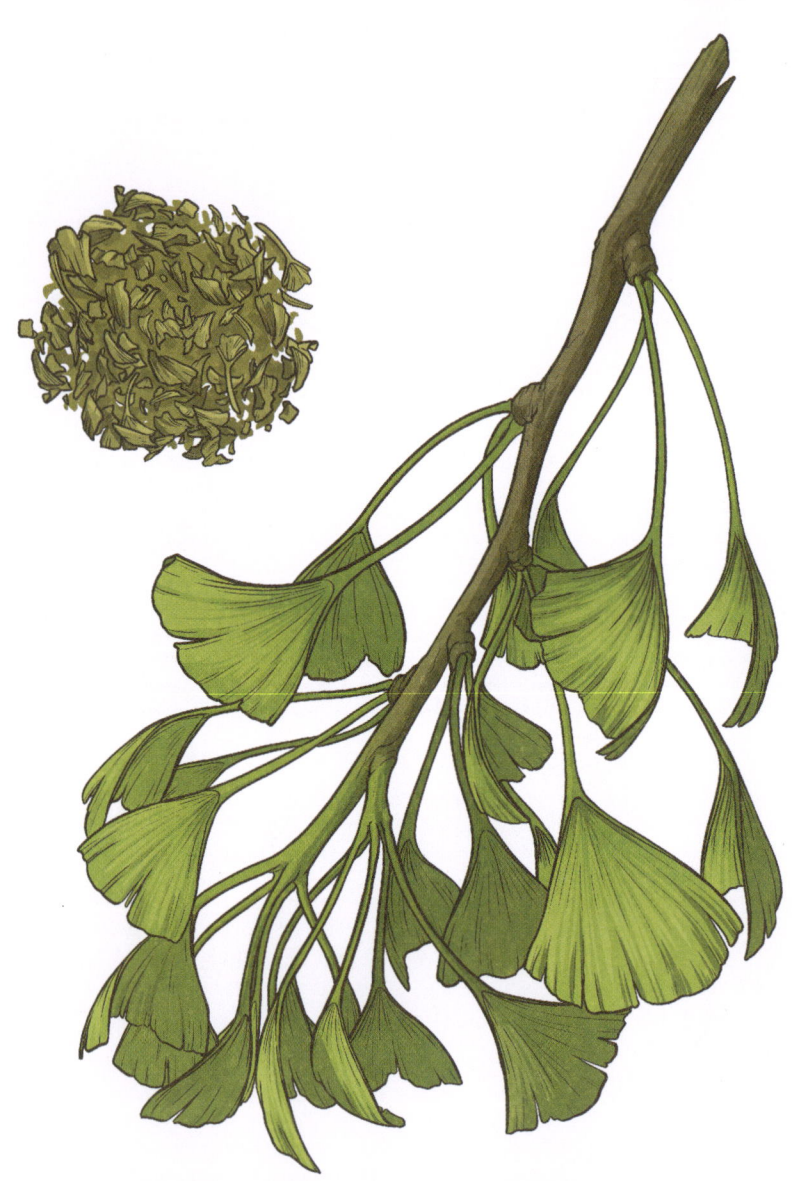

Ginkgo

Ginkgo biloba
Other name(s): maidenhair tree

Ginkgo has a long history of treating poor circulation and memory. It increases blood flow to the brain and limbs while strengthening the blood vessels, reducing clotting, and enhancing capillary circulation. Studies show potential benefits for senile dementia and depression in the elderly, and it may delay mental deterioration in the early stages of Alzheimer's disease. Due to its antioxidant properties, it can also be beneficial for the lungs, helping with cases of chronic bronchitis or asthma. It is very useful for brain fog, forgetfulness, and mild depression and combines well with gotu kola, tulsi, or any mint (helpful since the ginkgo leaf tastes rather bland!). It is best used as a tea or a tincture.

PARTS USED: leaf

MEDICINAL USES: anti-inflammatory, antioxidant, cognitive enhancer, circulatory enhancer

SAFETY CONSIDERATIONS: It may cause some gastrointestinal upset and rare allergic reactions. Use caution with circulatory disorders or chronic aspirin use.

REMEDIES: Clear the Fog Tea, Uplifting Nervous System Tonic, Lemon Verbena Refresher

TIP: Start with small doses to assess tolerance—some people are quite sensitive to ginkgo.

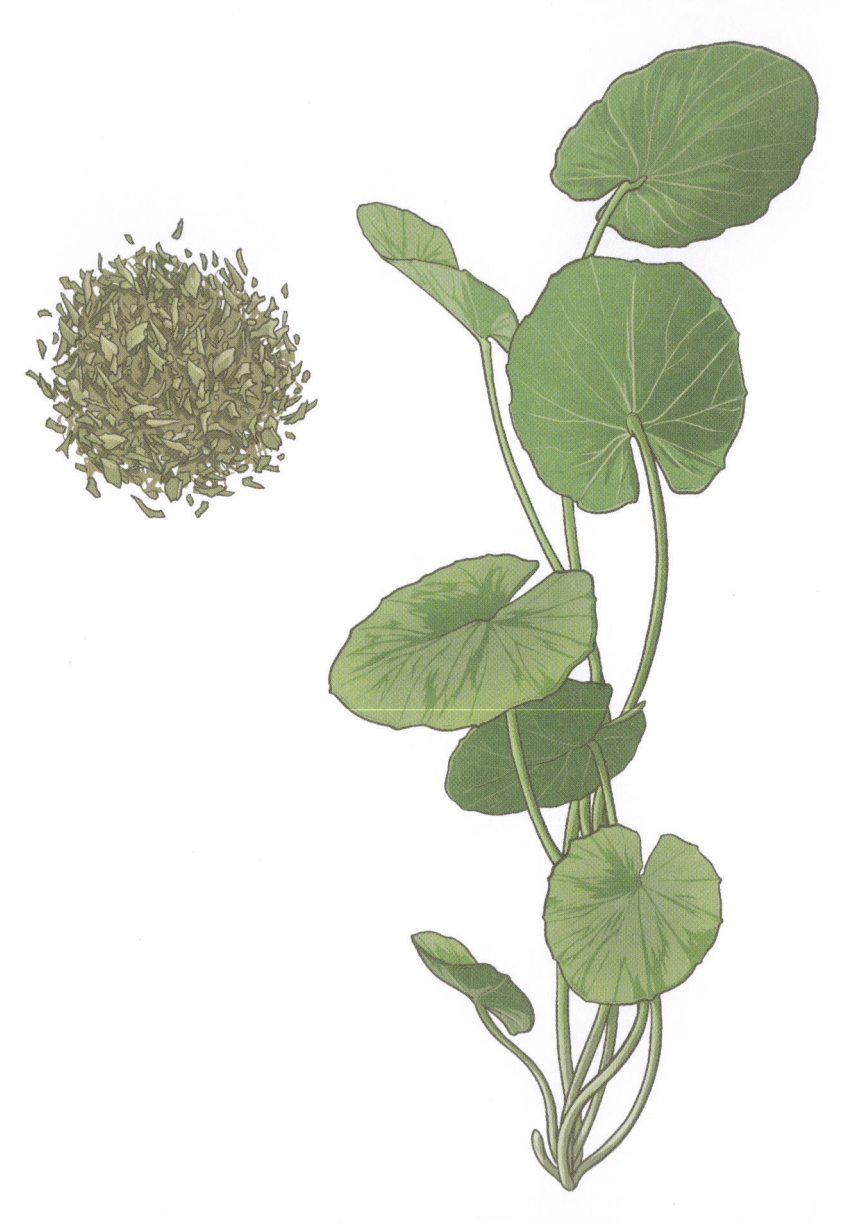

Gotu Kola

Centella asiatica
Other name(s): *Ji xue cao* (Chinese), *Brahmi* (Ayurveda)

Gotu kola is a cooling, spicy, and fragrant herb. In Chinese medicine, it belongs to the "herbs that clear heat and remove toxicity"—addressing fever and hot, inflammatory conditions needing antibiotic-like properties. Ayurvedic medicine uses it as a nerve tonic to help with memory, anxiety, and depression. My teacher K. P. noted that both Brahmi (*Centella asiatic*) and Bacopa (*Bacopa monniera*) share the name "Brahmi" in India, making ancient texts unclear, though both target the brain and nerves. Specifically it is useful in blends for memory and brain fog. It is best used as a tea or a tincture.

PARTS USED: whole plant, primarily aerial parts

MEDICINAL USES: anti-inflammatory, adaptogen, analgesic, wound-healing, diuretic, mild laxative, circulatory enhancer, antiseptic

SAFETY CONSIDERATIONS: Use cautiously during pregnancy due to its emmenagogue effect.

REMEDIES: Bone Strength Tea, Clear the Fog Tea, Lemon Verbena Refresher

TIP: Try this solo as a tea and see what effects you notice!

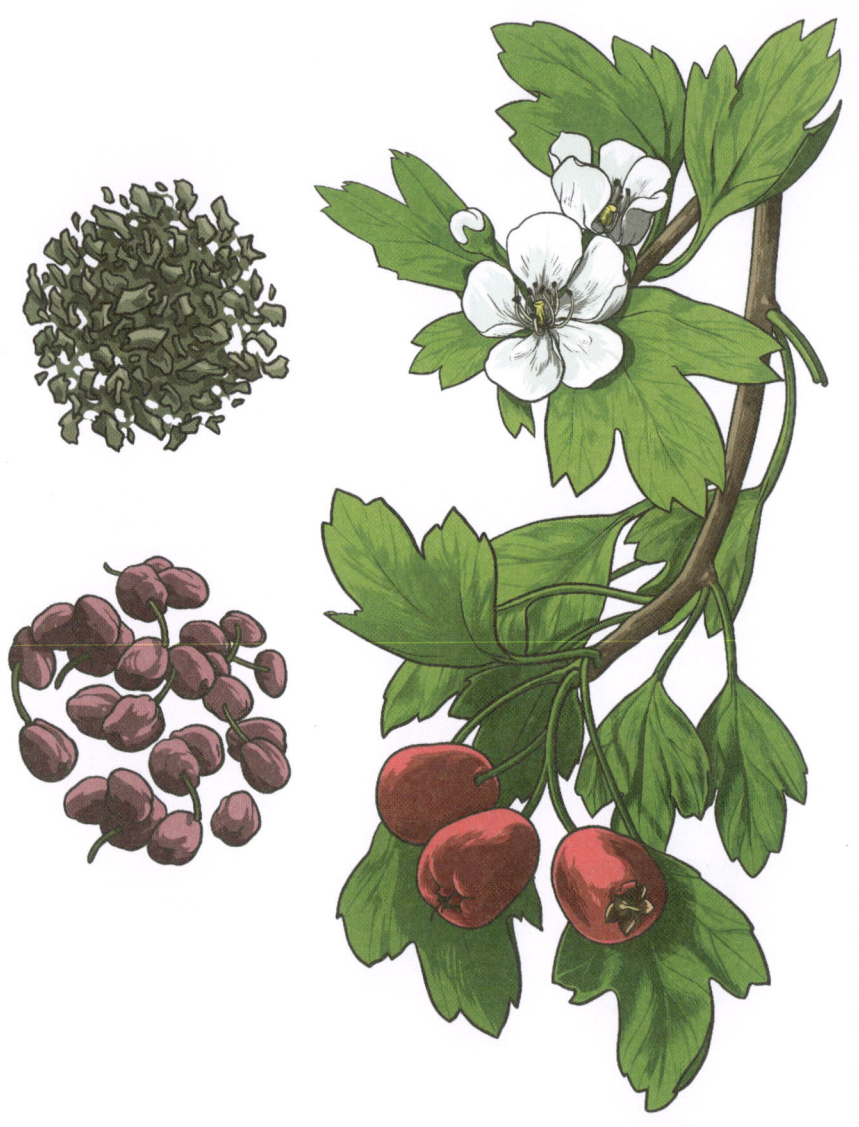

Hawthorn

Crataegus spp.
Other name(s): may, mayblossom, whitethorn,
hagthorn, ladies' meat

The hawthorn tree carries a long medicinal and sacred history.
Called mayblossom for its white flowers (with an off-putting smell to
some), it blooms in May. Uses include leaves, flowers, and berries.
The tree bears thorns ranging from small to intensely long. One
Pacific Northwest species (*C. monogyna*) spreads invasively via
birds eating and distributing seeds—wonderful for herbalists, but
challenging for homeowners! The berries provide cardiovascular
strengthening, supporting function and maintaining healthy venous
structure. This plant serves both the physical and the energetic
heart—addressing cardiovascular complaints plus grief, heartache,
depression, and sadness. Flowers and leaves soothe the nervous
system. The berry is best used as a decoction or tincture. The leaf
and flower are best used as an infusion.

PARTS USED: flowers, leaves,
twigs, berries

MEDICINAL USES: antioxidant,
cardiotonic, nutritious, astringent, diuretic

SAFETY CONSIDERATIONS:
Use with caution in combination
with heart medications.

REMEDIES: Herbal Iron Syrup,
Cholesterol Helper Tea, Warm
Me Up Tea, Healthy Heart Tea,
Healing Heart Syrup, Cold
Kicking Vinegar (optional addi-
tion), Lemon Verbena Refresher,
Long Life Oxymel.

TIP: Fresh berries make excellent
tinctures and cordials if you can
harvest them—otherwise dried
herbs work beautifully.

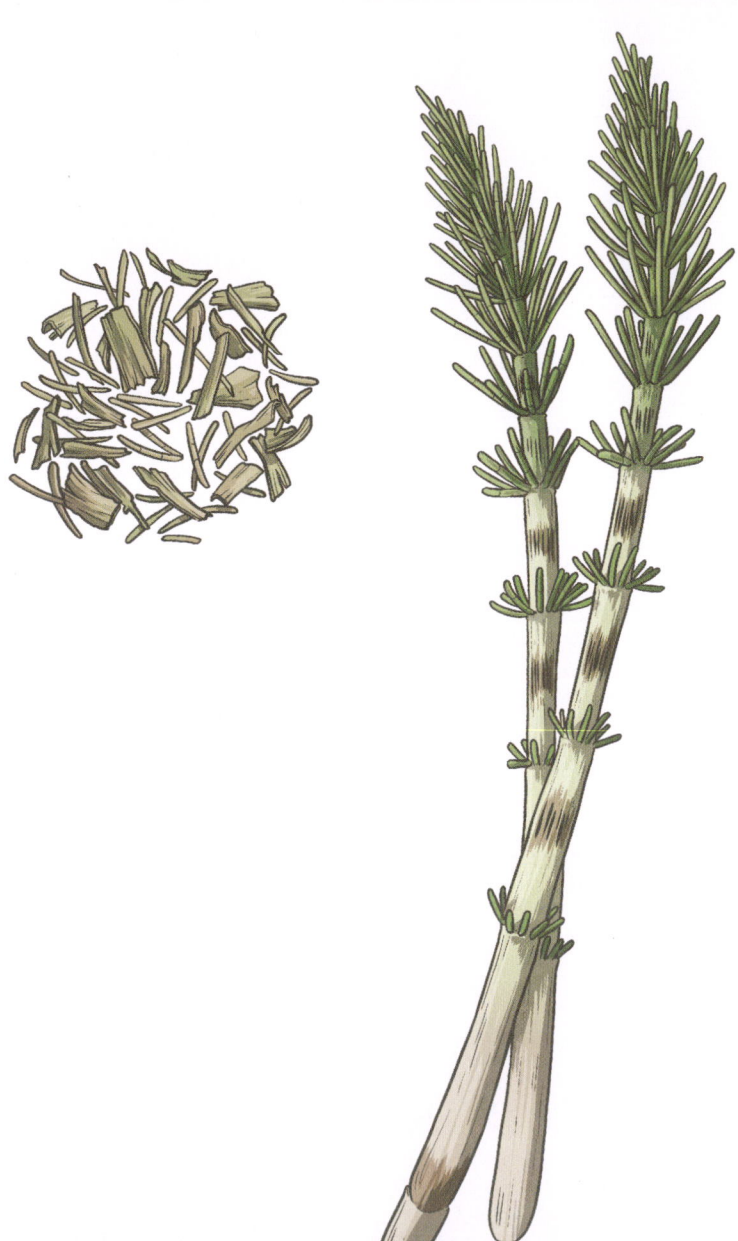

Horsetail

Equisetum arvense
Other name(s): shavegrass, bottlebrush, puzzle plant

This funny plant resembles a toilet brush popping from the ground in early spring! Harvest the tops just before they open completely to reveal the bottle brush. It's bland, slightly sweet, cooling, and drying. It's also high in iron, silicon, vitamin A, magnesium, manganese, chromium, calcium, potassium, and more, which makes it an excellent plant for the hair, skin, bones, nails, cartilage, and tissues of the body. I first learned that the Salish tribes in the Pacific Northwest eat the horsetail shoots in early spring from Elise Krohn in probably 2011; she has a lovely book about Northwest plants and speaks of native use and food as medicine. As a diuretic, horsetail tones and astringes the urinary system. It also works topically in washes for skin and hair. It is best used as an infusion.

PARTS USED: tops in spring, just before opening

MEDICINAL USES: diuretic, astringent, wound healing, helpful for tissue health, antibacterial, antispasmodic

SAFETY CONSIDERATIONS: Any diuretic consumed in large amounts should be used with caution, as it can drain essential minerals.

REMEDIES: Bye-Bye Bloat Tea, Bone Strength Tea, Shiny Happy Hair Tea, Flaky Scalp Hair Rinse, Long Life Oxymel

TIP: Steep for 15 minutes or several hours—its bland taste allows very long steeping without bitterness!

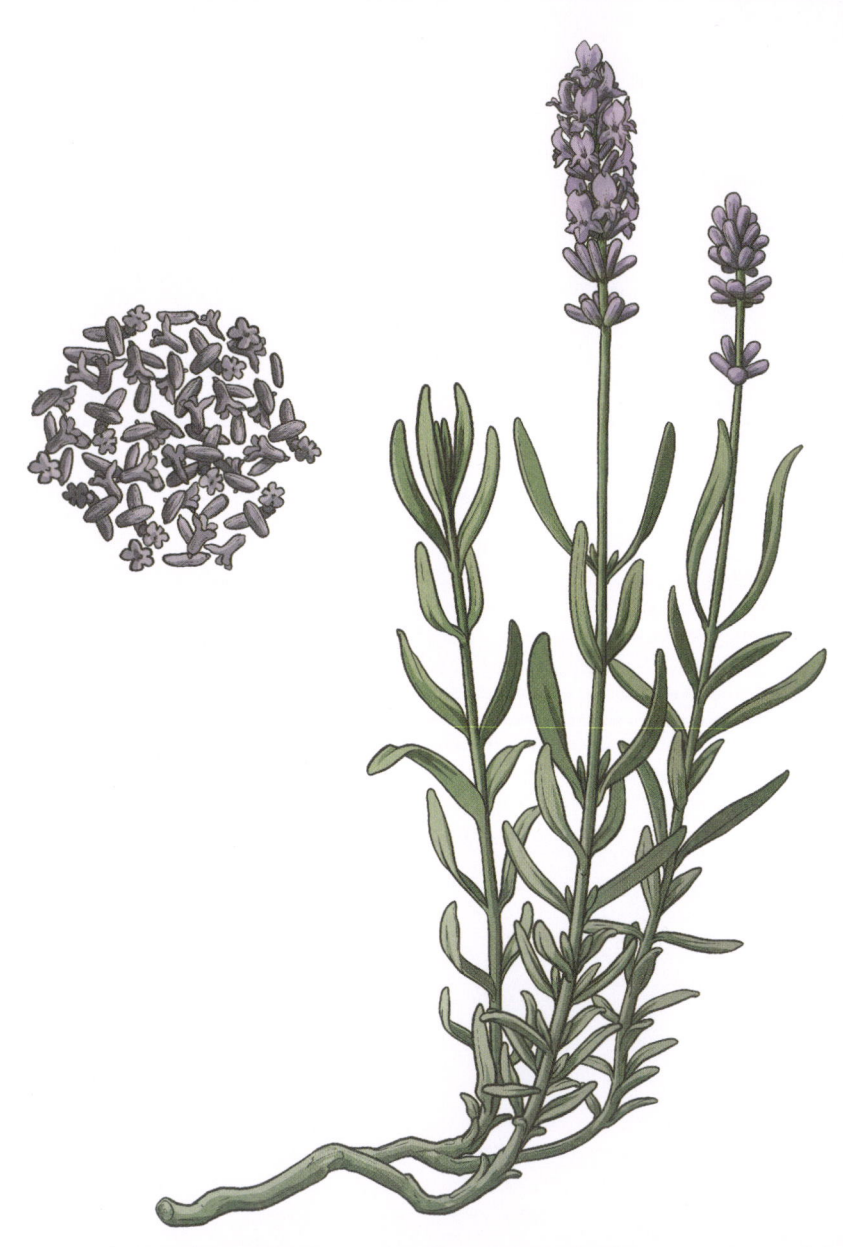

25

Lavender

Lavandula angustifolia (other species can be used, but this predominates)
Other name(s): none commonly used

Lavender's familiar scent has served people throughout Europe and the West for ages. The scent is herbaceous, and the flowers taste bitter. It is aromatic, cooling, and drying. Lavender stimulates circulation, calms the mind, reduces anxiety, and helps with pain and infection. As a mild sedative, it relaxes the mind and body into sleep. It is also a well-known burn aid. It is best used as tea or tincture, and it can also be used topically in washes, baths, and essential oils.

PARTS USED: flowers

MEDICINAL USES: anti-inflammatory, carminative, mild sedative, relaxant, mild antidepressant, wound healing

SAFETY CONSIDERATIONS: Use cautiously during pregnancy due to its emmenagogue effects.

REMEDIES: Acne Healing Vinegar, Passionflower Tincture (optional addition), Mugwort Healing Liniment, Herbal Foot Soak, Beautiful Skin Herbal Facial Steam, Get Back to Sleep Tincture, Jaw Clench Relief Poultice, The BEST Bug Spray (essential oil option), Let the Sun In Tea, Floral Herbal Toner, Herbal Skin Oil, Stress Relief Tea, Flaky Scalp Hair Rinse (essential oil option)

TIP: Grow lavender for fragrant dried bunches around the house, then use the buds for drawer sachets, dream pillows, or tea.

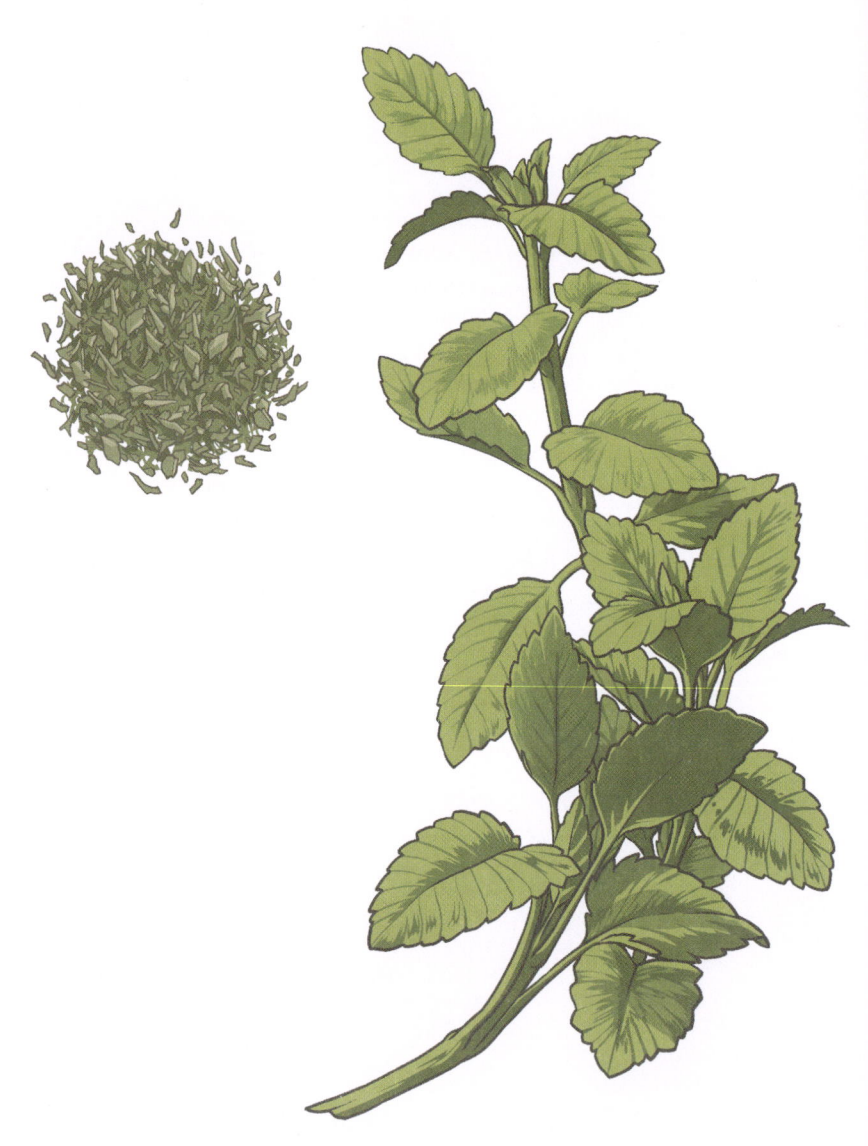

26

Lemon Balm

Melissa officinalis
Other name(s): melissa, sweet balm

Lemon balm is one of the most beloved herbs! It is sweet, slightly sour, aromatic, and warming. Mint-family herbs like lemon balm share calming properties and make delightful porch plants for multiple uses (flavoring water, adding to salads, drying for tea). Beyond taste, it excels as an aid for anxiety and eases digestive issues, such as upset stomach, bloating, or loss of appetite. It benefits those who are restless, agitated, or have heart palpitations or hypertension. Ryan Drum introduced its use for hyperthyroidism (fitting, as this condition often presents these characteristics). It works as a mild antidepressant too. Clinical trials show lavender cream reduces cold sore healing time significantly when used for herpes (viral infection). It is best used as an infusion or tincture.

PARTS USED: aerial parts

MEDICINAL USES: nervous system tonic, calming sedative, antispasmodic, antiviral, antioxidant

SAFETY CONSIDERATIONS: Use caution when used for hypothyroidism. It is contraindicated during pregnancy due to its emmenagogue effect.

REMEDIES: Acne Healing Vinegar, Anxie-Tea, Kick That Cold Sore Tea, Healthy Heart Tea, Fertili-Tea, Uplifting Nervous System Tonic, PMS Relief Tea, Floral Herbal Toner

TIP: Fresh lemon balm makes a delightful sun tea—fill a jar with leaves, add water, and steep in sunlight.

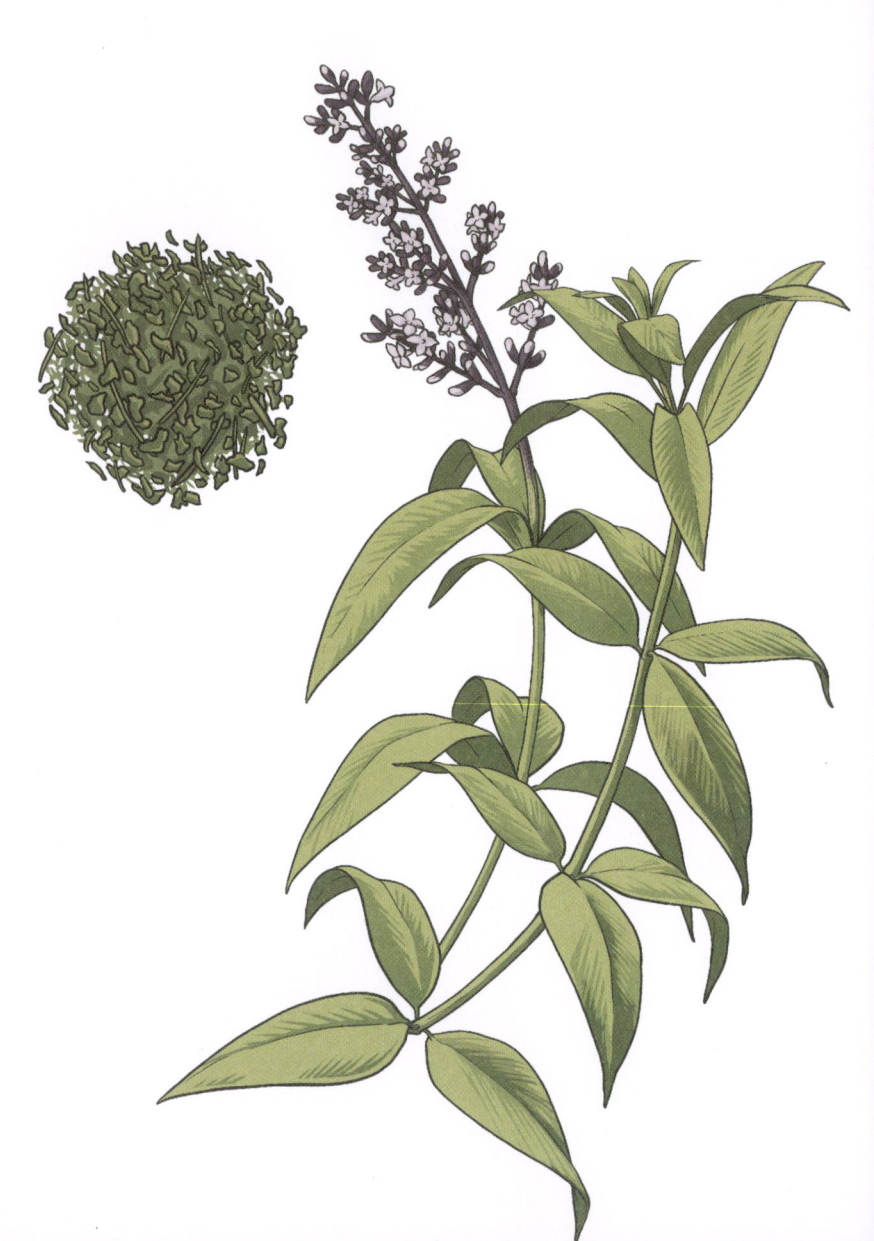

27

Lemon Verbena

Aloysia citrodora
Other name(s): lemon beebrush

This lovely, fragrant, leafy South American plant sometimes gets confused with lemon balm (probably because both have "lemon" in the name), but they represent different plant families (Lemon verbena: *Verbenaceae*; lemon balm: mint family *Lamiaceae*). Medicinally its uses are similar to lemon balm, but it is sweeter and gentler. It contains many volatile oils such as citral, cineole, limonene, and geraniol. It can be used for blends to calm, help with digestion, and lift the spirit. It is best used as an infusion.

PARTS USED: leaves

MEDICINAL USES: mild sedative, mild antidepressant, carminative, antispasmodic

SAFETY CONSIDERATIONS: none noted

REMEDIES: Anxie-Tea, Lemon Verbena Refresher, PMS Relief Tea, Stress Relief Tea (optional swap)

TIP: Dried leaves maintain fragrance for months—add to potpourri or drawer sachets between uses.

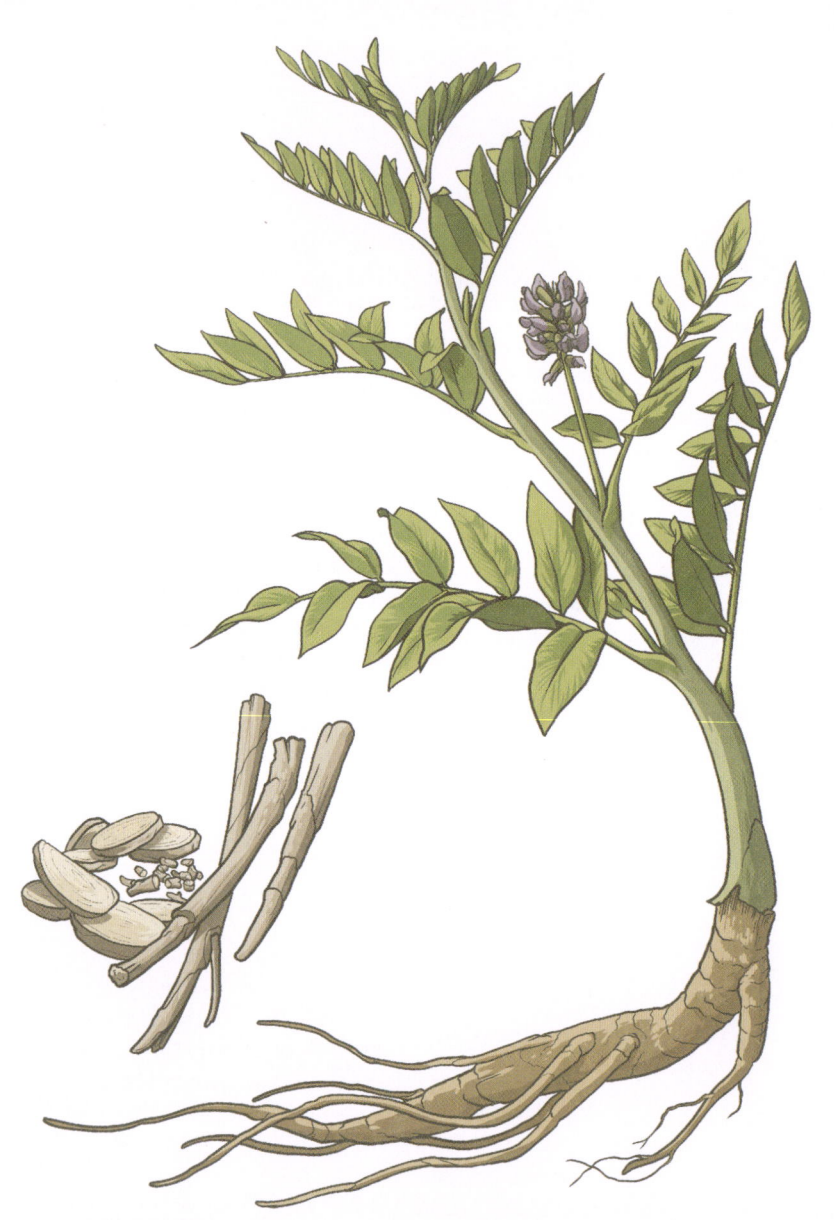

Licorice

Glycyrrhiza glabra
Other name(s): sweetwood

True licorice differs greatly from candy versions! It tastes sweet and woody, but also slightly bitter. Herbal medicine practice across the world's cultures has used licorice for centuries. In Chinese medicine, it reduces toxicity and harmonizes with other herbs. Its demulcent qualities soothe sore throats, stomachs, and intestines. As an adaptogen, it helps the body modulate stressors, reduce inflammation, and affect hormone balance. Clinically versatile! It is best used as a long infusion, decoction, or tincture.

PARTS USED: root

MEDICINAL USES: antispasmodic, anti-inflammatory, laxative, expectorant, antibacterial, antifungal, adaptogen

SAFETY CONSIDERATIONS: Licorice can raise blood pressure. Those with hypertension should work with healthcare professionals (some Chinese medicine dosing actually lowers it with proper understanding). Use caution with liver and kidney disorders due to choleretic action (bile stimulation). Toxicity symptoms include hypertension, headaches, and vertigo—usually from high, frequent doses.

REMEDIES: Dry Those Drips Tea, Bone Strength Tea, Warm Me Up Tea, Kick That Cold Sore Tea, Easy Mover Tea, Cough Syrup, Dry Cough Tea, Tummy Ease Tea, Root Beer Syrup, Healthy Heart Tea, Women's Rooted Tea, Cool Me Down Hot Flash Tincture, Happy Lungs Tea, Lymph Mover Tea, Stop the Sweats Tincture, Restless Legs Relief Tea, Stress Less Herbal Chai, Sore Throat Soother

TIP: Licorice root is quite different from the candy—it has a honey-like sweetness that's naturally soothing. Try adding a pinch to your tea or tasting it on its own to experience the unique flavor of this magical root!

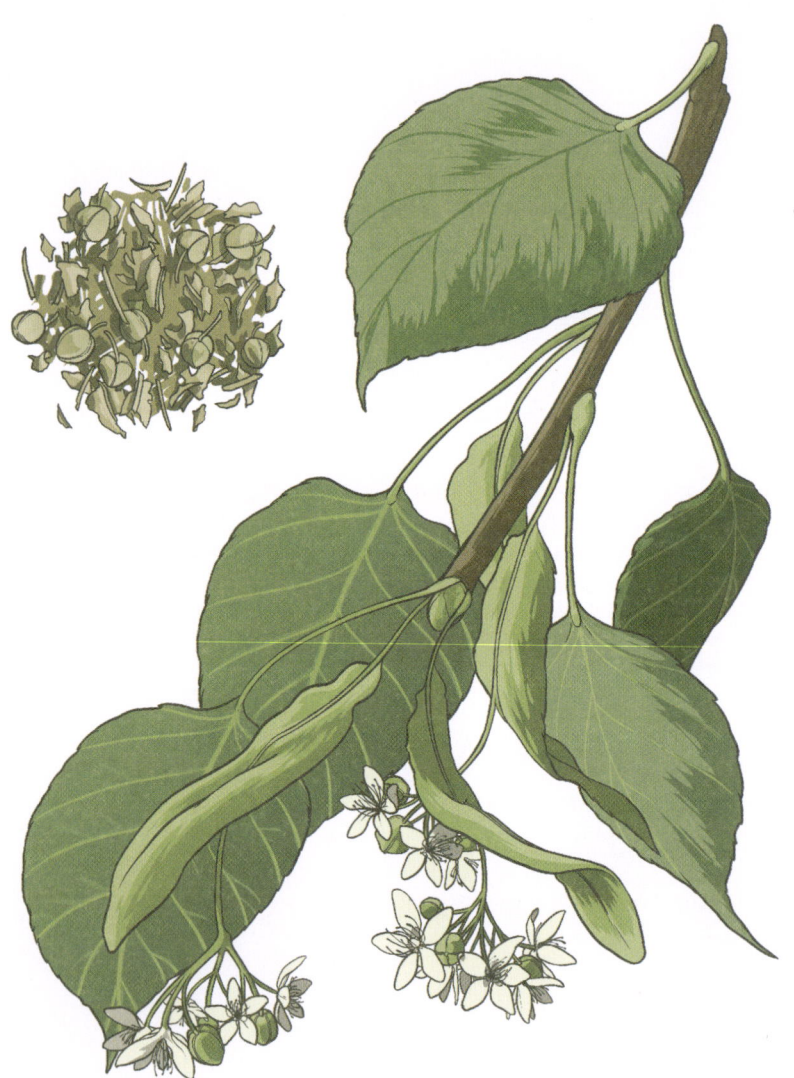

Linden

Tilia spp.
Other name(s): lime tree, teil tree, basswood, bast tree, spoonwood

In spring the Linden produces whitish-green, slightly sweet flowers with a feathery, wispy appearance—perfect fairy dwellings! The fresh flowers smell wonderfully sweet. Known as a relaxing diaphoretic, Linden can induce sweat at infection onset or during respiratory illness. It also helps with tense muscles and stress. It can provide a soothing tea for tender, depressed states or overactive nervous systems needing calming (combines beautifully with oat buds in an overnight infusion—drink several cups the next day). It is best used as an infusion or tincture.

PARTS USED: flower and leaves

MEDICINAL USES: diaphoretic, diuretic, antispasmodic, antidepressant

SAFETY CONSIDERATIONS: none noted

REMEDIES: Linden Oat Straw Infusion for a Broken Heart, Healthy Heart Tea

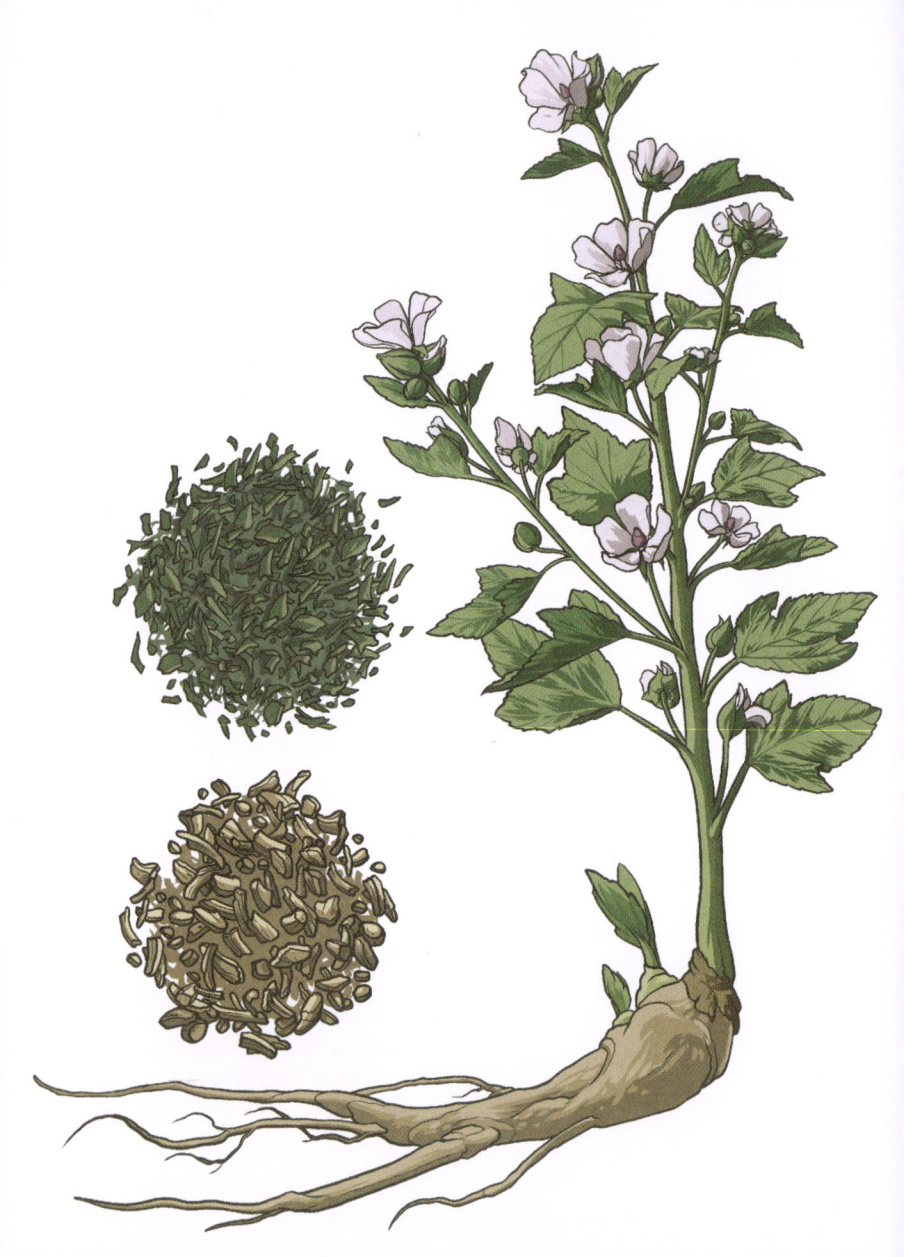

Marshmallow

Althea officinalis
Other name(s): white mallow, sweetweed

Marshmallow provides sweet, cooling, mucilaginous qualities filled with polysaccharides, pectin, sugars, calcium, and trace minerals. The root most commonly soothes mucous membranes—the lungs after respiratory illness or the digestive system. It can treat acute respiratory conditions due to its anti-inflammatory properties, plus any internal imbalance needing moistening and cooling such as urinary tract issues. In recent years it has been discovered that the leaves and flowers offer similar benefits—how wonderful to use the whole plant! Leaves and flowers prove very nutritive. The root is used best as a cold infusion or tincture; leaves are best used as a hot infusion. Marshmallow makes excellent external washes for inflammatory skin concerns.

PARTS USED: root, leaves, and flowers

MEDICINAL USES: mucilaginous, antispasmodic, anti-inflammatory, nutritious, mildly diuretic

SAFETY CONSIDERATIONS: Oral drugs or herbs taken simultaneously with marshmallow may have delayed absorption due to mucilage content.

REMEDIES: Reflux Relief Tea, Cold Infused Marshmallow Root for Acid Reflux, Blood Sugar Stabilizer Tea, Easy Mover Tea, Cough Syrup, Dry Cough Tea, Cool Down and Rehydrate Tea, Soothing Tea for Nausea, Happy Lungs Tea, Rehydrating Tea for the Runs, Sore Throat Soother, Herbal Bath for Itchy Skin

TIP: Marshmallow leaves and flowers hold a special place in my heart—and they're very pretty. If you have the chance to try them fresh or dried as a tea, don't miss it!

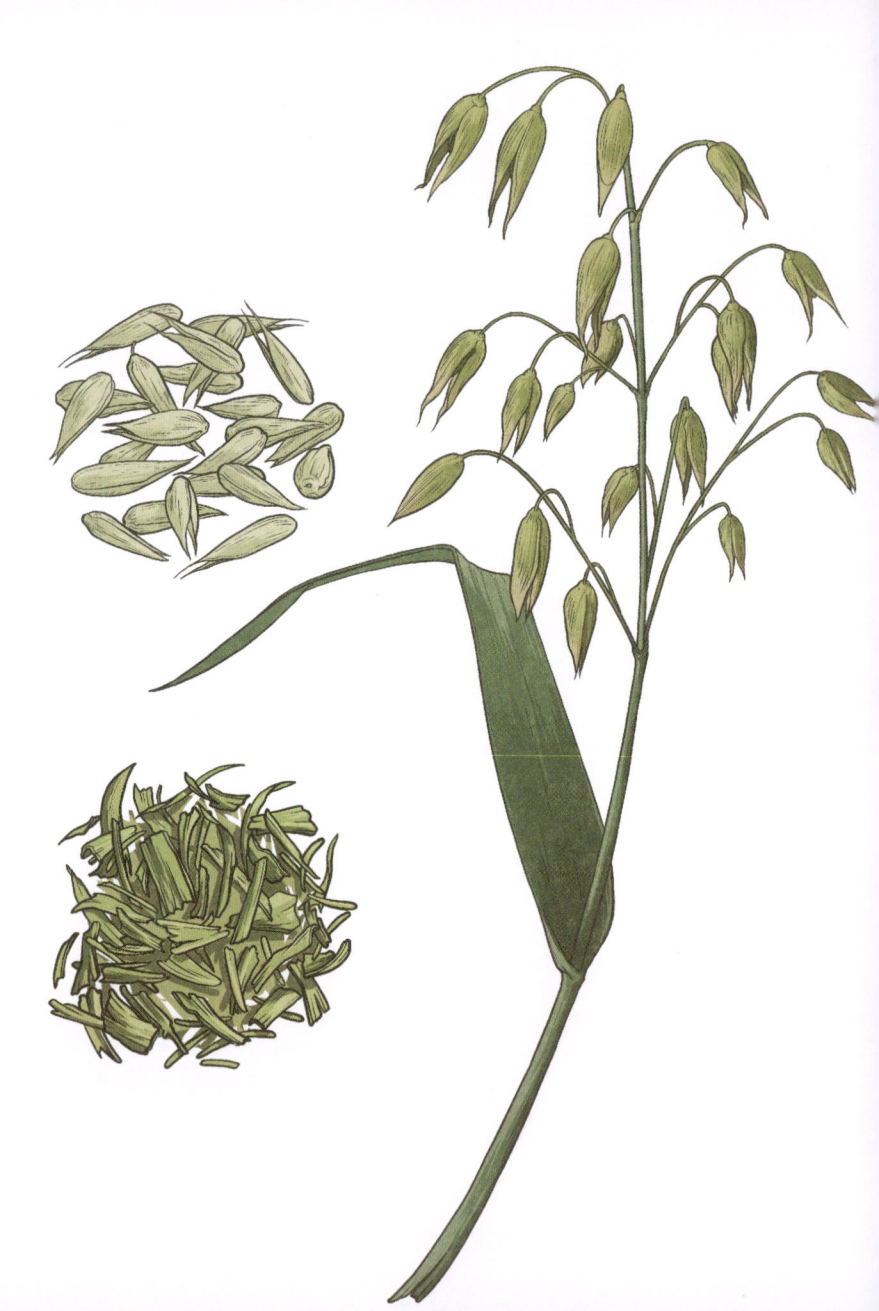

Milky Oat

Avena sativa
Other name(s): milky oat buds, oat buds, oat heads,
oat straw, oat grass

Milky oats have become an increasingly beloved herb over the years! Sweet, nutritious, and moistening—the oat grain from ripened seed provides high protein, while the plant offers magnesium, chromium, silicon, vitamin A, manganese, zinc, and B vitamins. This daily nutritious tonic addresses serious anxiety, restlessness, and exhaustion. Studies show it can relieve withdrawal symptoms from substances such as nicotine and opioids. It is best used as a long infusion or tincture from the fresh buds. Rolled oats (the processed, toasted, flattened oat groats we eat as oatmeal) can be eaten or used as a wash for your skin. Milky oat buds or straw can also be used in baths.

PARTS USED: milky oat seeds, or the shredded version called oat straw

MEDICINAL USES: nervous system tonic, sedative, nervine, nutritious

SAFETY CONSIDERATIONS: none noted

REMEDIES: Anxie-Tea, Arthritis Alleviation Tea, Bone Strength Tea, Uplifting Nervous System Tonic, Tummy Ease Tea, Daily Multivitamin Tea, Long Life Oxymel, Linden Oat Straw Infusion for a Broken Heart, Shiny Happy Hair Tea, Hangover Hydration Tea, Healthy Heart Tea, Hemmy Soothe Herbal Wash (optional addition), Fertili-Tea, Get to Sleep Tea, In-the-Mood Damiana Cordial, Mother's Nursing Blend, Pain Relieving Tea, PMS Relief Tea, Stress Relief Tea, Restless Leg Relief Tea

TIP: Fresh milky oat tincture is much more effective than the dry version. If you don't have access to the fresh version, drink the infusion daily.

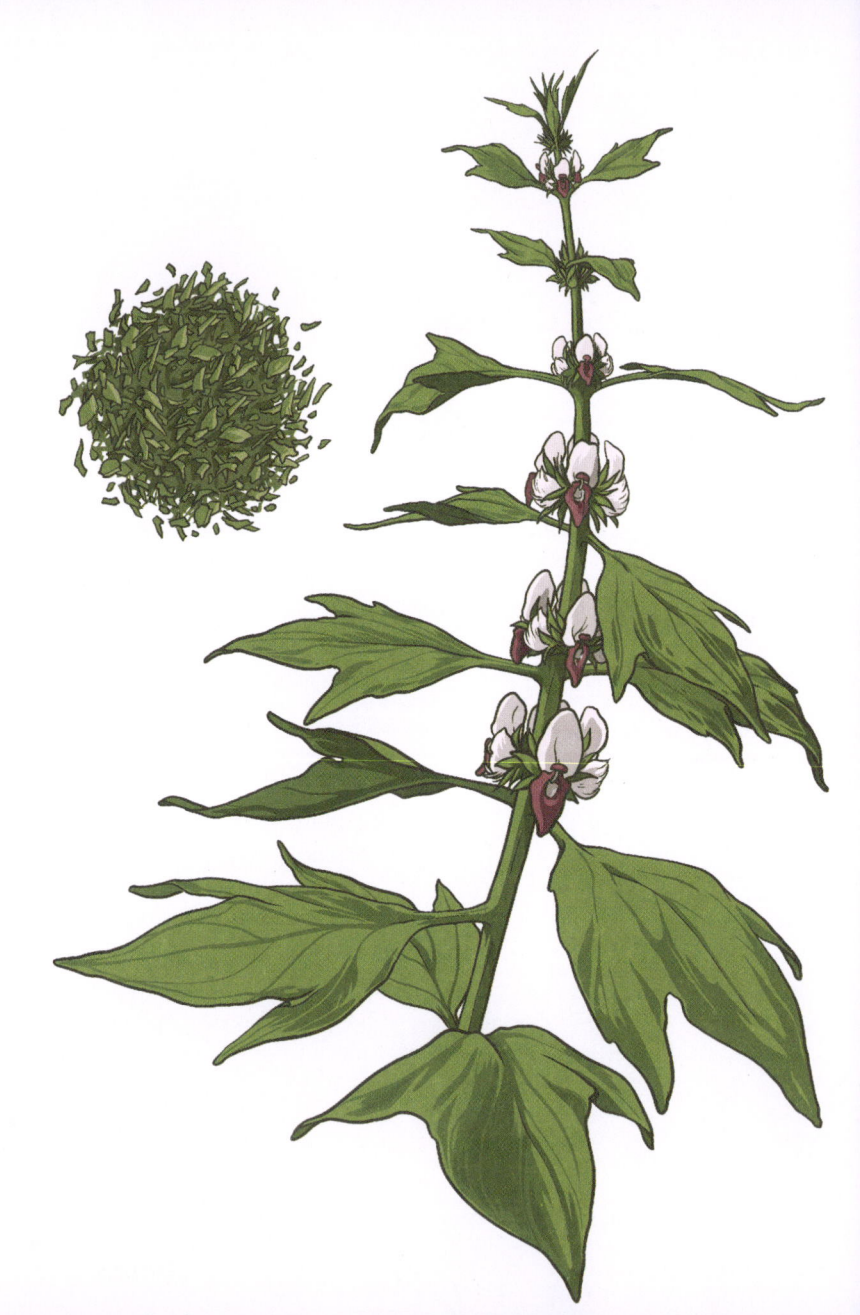

Motherwort

Leonurus cardiaca
Other name(s): lion's tail

Motherwort is a bitter, cool, and drying plant that is used for various emotional and gynecological issues, hence "motherwort" meaning "beneficial for the mother." The genus name, *Leonurus*, means a "lion's tail" in Greek, referencing the plant's appearance. It can be helpful for women's imbalances, including painful periods, stress, postpartum blood loss, and hemorrhaging. It can also address emotional PMS symptoms, such as anxiety, heart palpitations, insomnia, and irritability. It is best used as an infusion or tincture.

PARTS USED: aerial parts

MEDICINAL USES: women's tonic herb, diaphoretic, diuretic, antispasmodic, nervine, emmenagogue

SAFETY CONSIDERATIONS: It is contraindicated during pregnancy due to its emmenagogue effect.

REMEDIES: Cool Me Down Hot Flash Tincture, After Birth Rebalance Tea (optional addition)

TIP: This is another herb that can be taken on its own as a tincture for symptoms such as hot flashes, heart palpitations, and night sweats. It's quite bitter, so it's best diluted in a small amount of water.

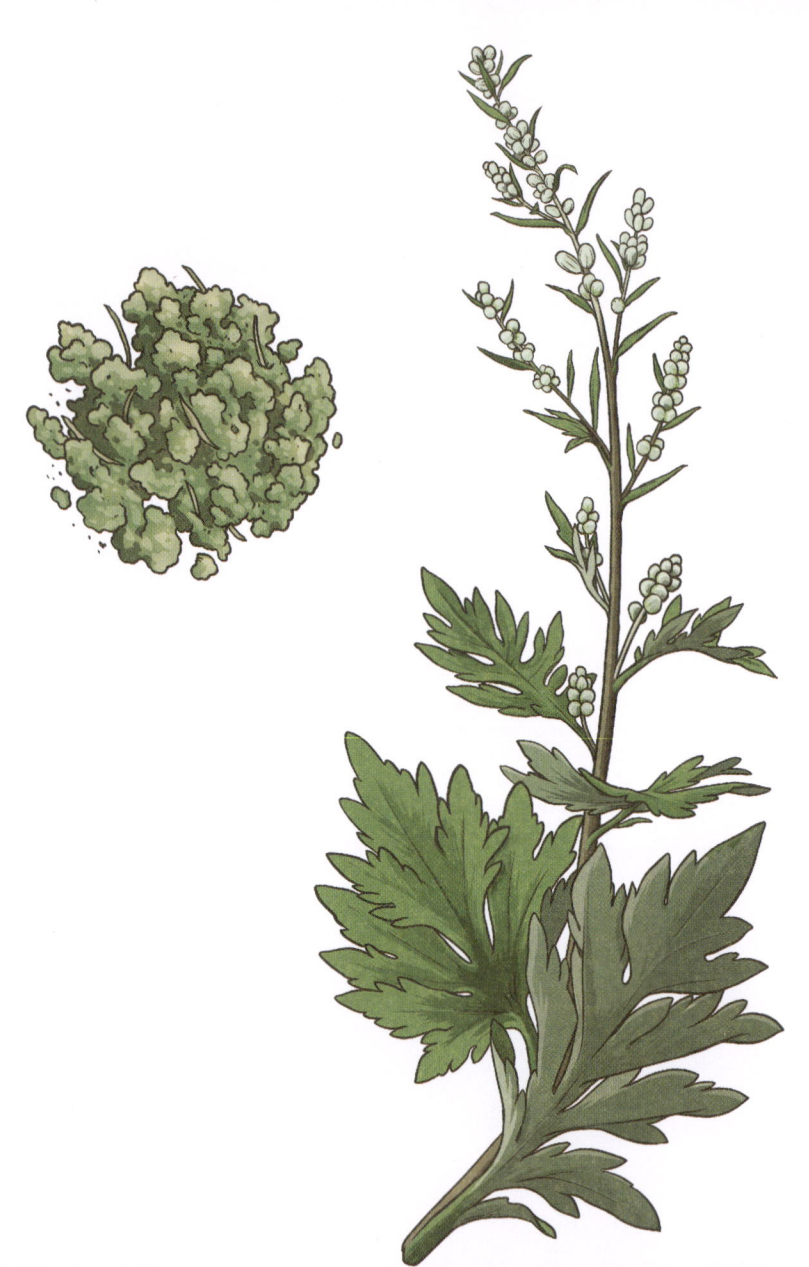

Mugwort

Artemisia vulgaris
Other name(s): St. John's plant

Mugwort grows tall with aromatic, bitter, spicy, warming qualities—and has a purple-green hue with white leaf undersides. The medieval nickname "St. John's plant" arose from a belief that John the Baptist wore bundles of it around his waist for protection from fatigue, wild beasts, and evil spirits. Medicinally it serves digestion as a bitter and helps bring on menstruation. East Asian bath houses commonly use mugwort washes to warm and tonify the uterus and for menstruation. Chinese medicine uses it for moxibustion—ground into cotton-candy texture and burned on acupuncture points. Ingested or placed near a pillow for dream work, it can bring on vivid dreams or help dream consciousness. It is best used as an infusion or tincture.

PARTS USED: aerial parts

MEDICINAL USES: bitter for digestion, antispasmodic, nervine, emmenagogue, diaphoretic

SAFETY CONSIDERATIONS: It is contraindicated during pregnancy due to its emmenagogue effect.

REMEDIES: Mugwort Healing Liniment, Dreamer's Cordial

TIP: This plant has one of the most captivating scents on the planet. If you encounter it in the wild, gently rub the leaves and inhale the aroma. It's truly otherworldly!

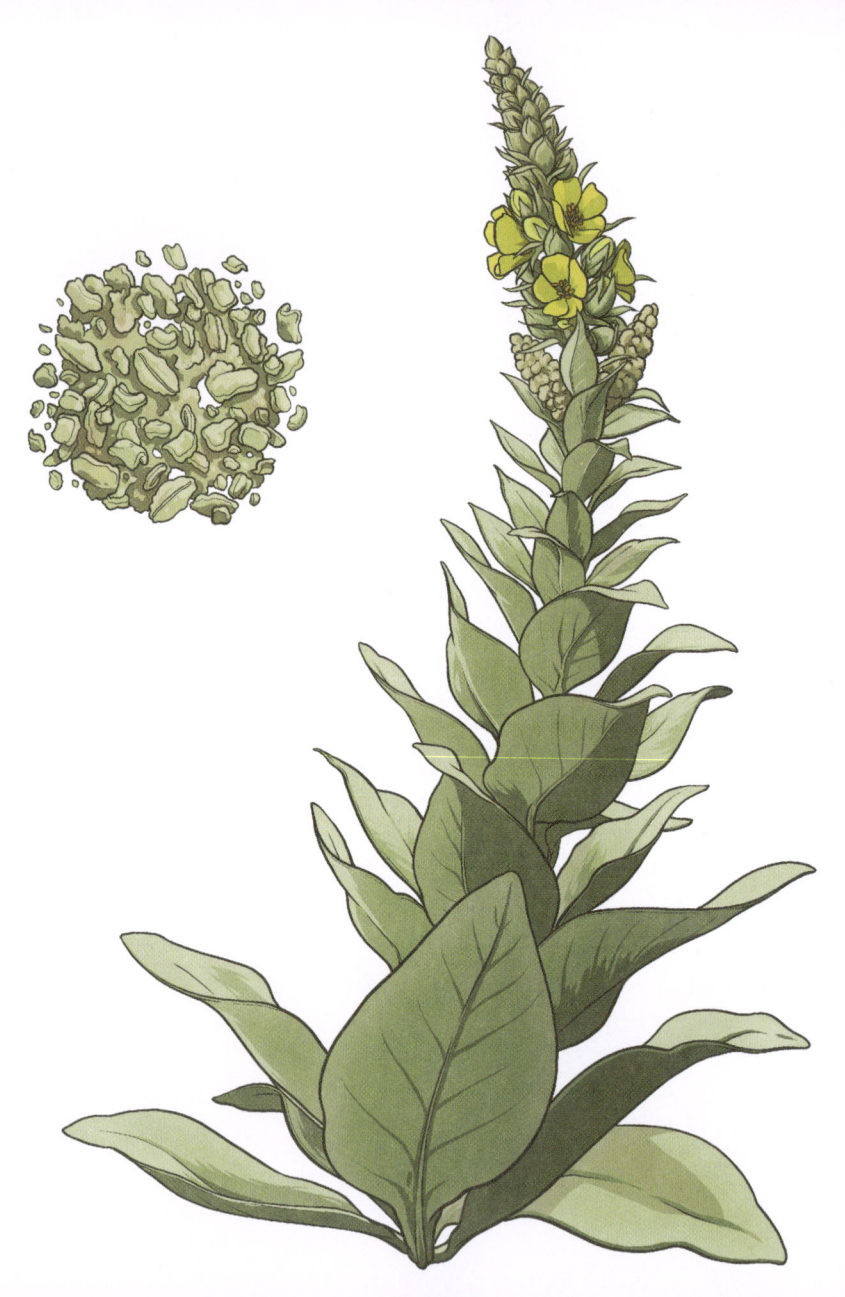

Mullein

Verbascum thapsus
Other name(s): our lady's candle, hag or hedge taper, candlewick plant, velvet plant, Aaron's rod, Jupiter's staff

Mullein stands tall at 4 to 5 feet, sometimes taller, with large, fuzzy light-green leaves and yellow flowers in dense, crowded spikes. Candle-referenced names reflect its blooming appearance—like a glowing candle. Historically used as a torch, its dried stalks were dipped in wax to burn as a "hag's taper" (use carefully if you want to recreate the effect!). Its leaves broadly treat respiratory illness, while its astringent and moistening effects soothe coughing, bronchitis, and wheezing. The flowers prove more demulcent, calming the nervous system and treating earaches or infections. It is best used as tea or tincture. The flowers are often made into an oil for earaches.

PARTS USED: leaves and flowers

MEDICINAL USES: demulcent, expectorant, astringent, anti-inflammatory, antibacterial

SAFETY CONSIDERATIONS: None noted

REMEDIES: Cough Syrup, Dry Cough Tea, Happy Lungs Tea, Lymph Mover Tea, Mullein Garlic Oil for Earache

TIP: Mullein leaves have tiny hairs that can irritate the esophagus, so it's generally best to use the dried form, which is typically well tolerated. If you prepare tea with fresh leaves, use a fine cloth over your strainer to help filter out as many of the hairs as possible.

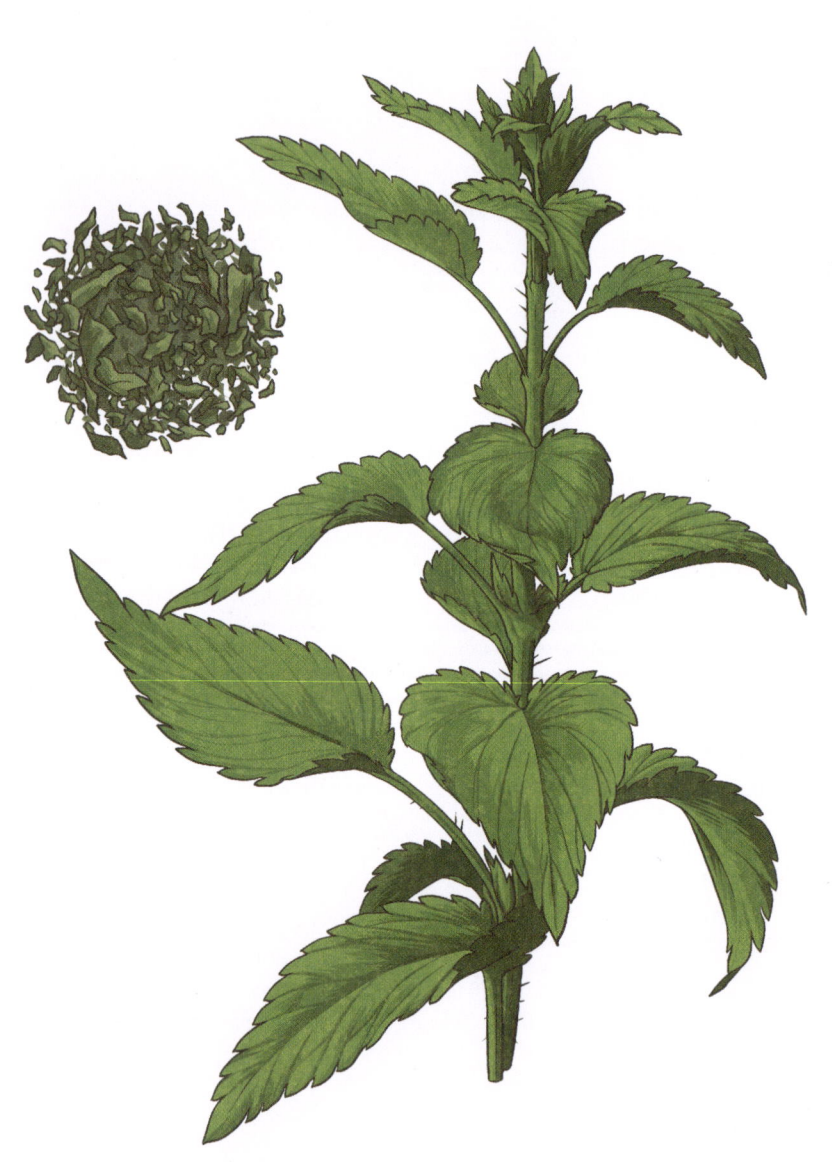

Nettle

Urtica dioica
Other name(s): stinging nettle

Stinging nettle provides incredible medicine to relieve arthritic pain and allergy symptoms. The plant leaf is lined with stingers, with tips breaking off when they contact the skin, releasing an array of compounds that bring relief to arthritic, cold, damp pain. The histamine reaction indicates a high quercetin content, which combats itchy eyes, runny nose, and sneezing. The leaf is best used as a cold infusion, as fresh or dried seeds, or in tincture form. Tincture or decoction is recommended for the root. Tops can be eaten fresh if blanched first.

PARTS USED: aerial tops (spring tips before buds appear), root, seed

MEDICINAL USES: astringent, diuretic, anti-inflammatory, nutritious

SAFETY CONSIDERATIONS: It is contraindicated in large doses during pregnancy due to its emmenagogue effect, though still beneficial and nutritious for pregnant women in moderate amounts.

REMEDIES: Dry Those Drips Tea, Cold Infusion Nettle Tea, Herbal Iron Syrup, Iron Tea, Arthritis Alleviation Tea, Bye-Bye Bloat Tea, Bone Strength Tea, Soothing Tummy Gummies (optional addition), Gentle Eczema Helper Tea, Long Life Oxymel, Shiny Happy Hair Tea, Daily Multivitamin Tea, Fertili-Tea, Mother's Nursing Blend, After Birth Rebalance Tea, Restless Leg Relief Tea

TIP: Gloves are highly recommended when working with nettle leaves—stings can affect sensitive people for a week!

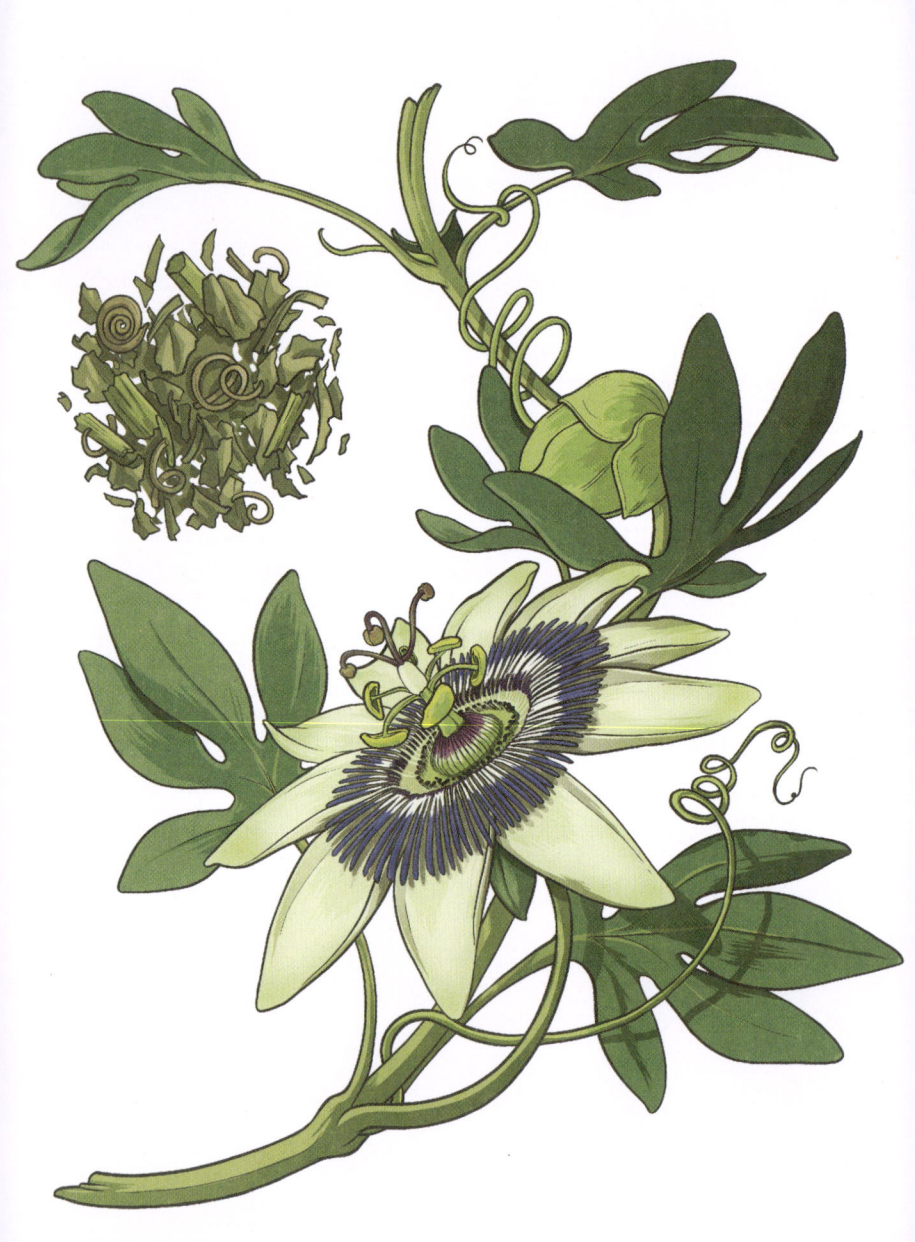

Passionflower

Passiflora incarnata
Other name(s): passion vine, maypop

Passionflower blooms look otherworldly! The flowers tend to be white and purple with curlicue vines (you'll find curls in the dried herb—delightful!). Cooling and possessing a slightly bitter aromatic scent, passionflower benefits those who are nervous, anxious, experiencing heart palpitations, have difficulty sleeping, have muscle spasms, or suffer from stress and anxiety. It is best used as an infusion or tincture.

PARTS USED: flowers (some stems and leaves)

MEDICINAL USES: antispasmodic, nervine, sedative, anti-inflammatory, pain reliever, anxiolytic (anxiety reducer)

SAFETY CONSIDERATIONS: Use with caution in early pregnancy due to its uterine stimulating effect. Be careful with barbiturates as it may enhance the sedative effect.

REMEDIES: Anxie-Tea, Passionflower Tincture for Anxiety, Get Back to Sleep Tincture, Stress Relief Tea

TIP: Many ornamental passionflowers aren't edible—ensure correct species identification before harvesting.

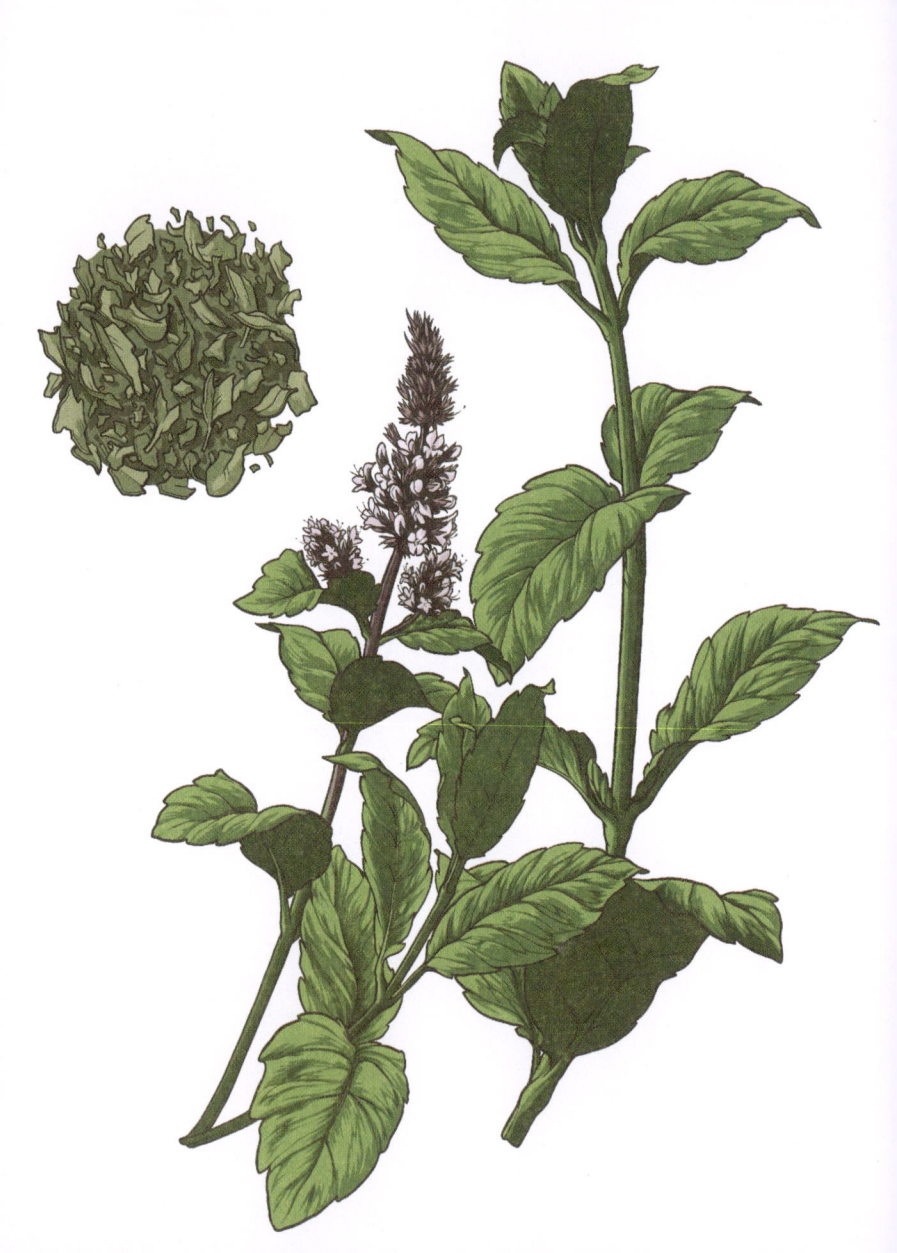

37

Peppermint

Mentha piperita
Other name(s): None commonly used

Peppermint offers familiar sweet, cooling, drying qualities with renowned aromatic properties. Excellent for general indigestion, nausea, and gas. For cold/flu symptoms, it provides relief as tea or as steam for sinus congestion and headaches—useful for all headache types. As diaphoretic, peppermint helps the body sweat and cool during fever. As cholagogue, it aids in bile release while supporting liver, gallbladder, and the digestive system. It works as bug repellent too! Menthol, peppermint oil's chief constituent, commonly appears in pain topicals—it opens pores, allowing herb penetration (Chinese medicine uses this to help other formulas penetrate). It is best used as an infusion or tincture.

PARTS USED: leaf

MEDICINAL USES: antispasmodic, carminative, diaphoretic, anti-inflammatory, diuretic, cholagogue

SAFETY CONSIDERATIONS: Though peppermint has emmenagogue effects, it's safe for pregnant people with morning sickness when used moderately.

REMEDIES: Dry Those Drips Tea, Iron Tea (optional addition), Arthritis Alleviation Tea (optional addition), Bone Strength Tea, Clear the Fog Tea, Herbalist's Bug Bit Poultice, Cold Kicker Tea (essential oil), Stuffy Head Sinus Steam, Dry Cough Tea, Tummy Ease Tea

TIP: Peppermint provides the most intense mint aromatics, but other mints can be substituted with similar effects!

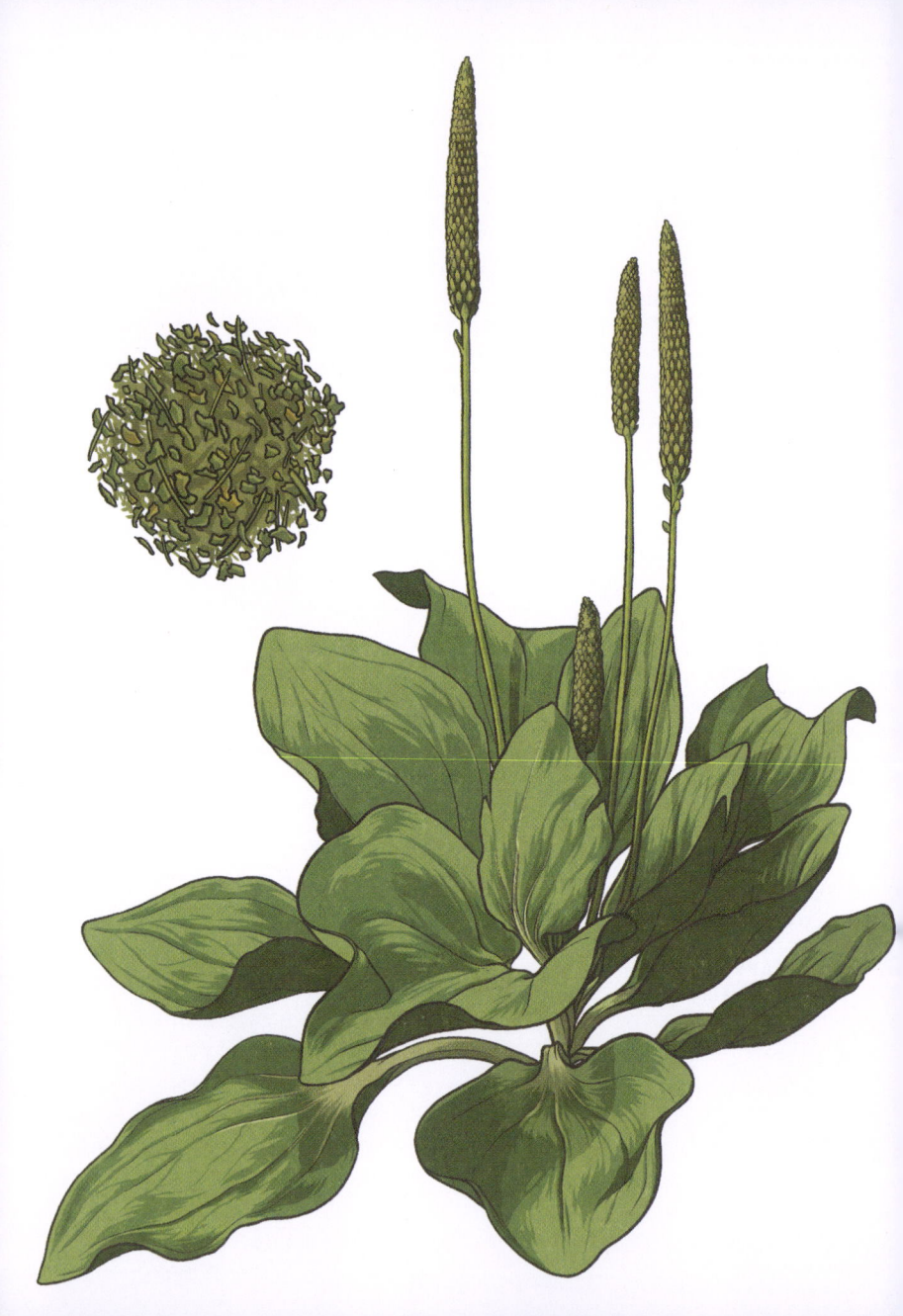

38

Plantain

Plantago lanceolata, P. major
Other name(s): lance leaf plantain, narrowleaf English
plantain, buckhorn plantain (*all Plantago lanceolata),*
broad leaf plantain (*P. major*)

Plantain grows as a cooling, drying weed offering wonderful remedies. The Pacific Northwest features two main species: broadleaf
and narrowleaf plantain (their names describe their appearance!).
This plant's medicine became clear to me during an outdoor herbalist training when relentless mosquito bites made focus impossible.
Another herbalist demonstrated the spit poultice method (chew
and apply to the bite)—the instant relief revealed herbal medicine's
amazing power! Plantain abounds in minerals (very nutritious), provides mucilaginous properties, helps inflammation, and tonifies the
urinary tract. It also moves lymph and expectorates phlegm while
nourishing lung tissue. It soothes the digestive tract beautifully.

PARTS USED: leaf

MEDICINAL USES: antibacterial, antiseptic, diuretic,
anti-inflammatory, nutritious,
astringent, wound healing,
expectorant

SAFETY CONSIDERATIONS:
none noted

REMEDIES: Reflux Relief Tea,
Gentle Liver Tonic Tea for Acne,
Herbalist's Bug Bite Poultice,
Lymph Mover Tea (optional
addition), Calendula Comfrey
Skin Salve

TIP: This also makes a beautiful
green herbal oil. It can be used
on its own as a massage oil or
made into a salve for various skin
needs, including burns, scrapes,
and other minor abrasions.

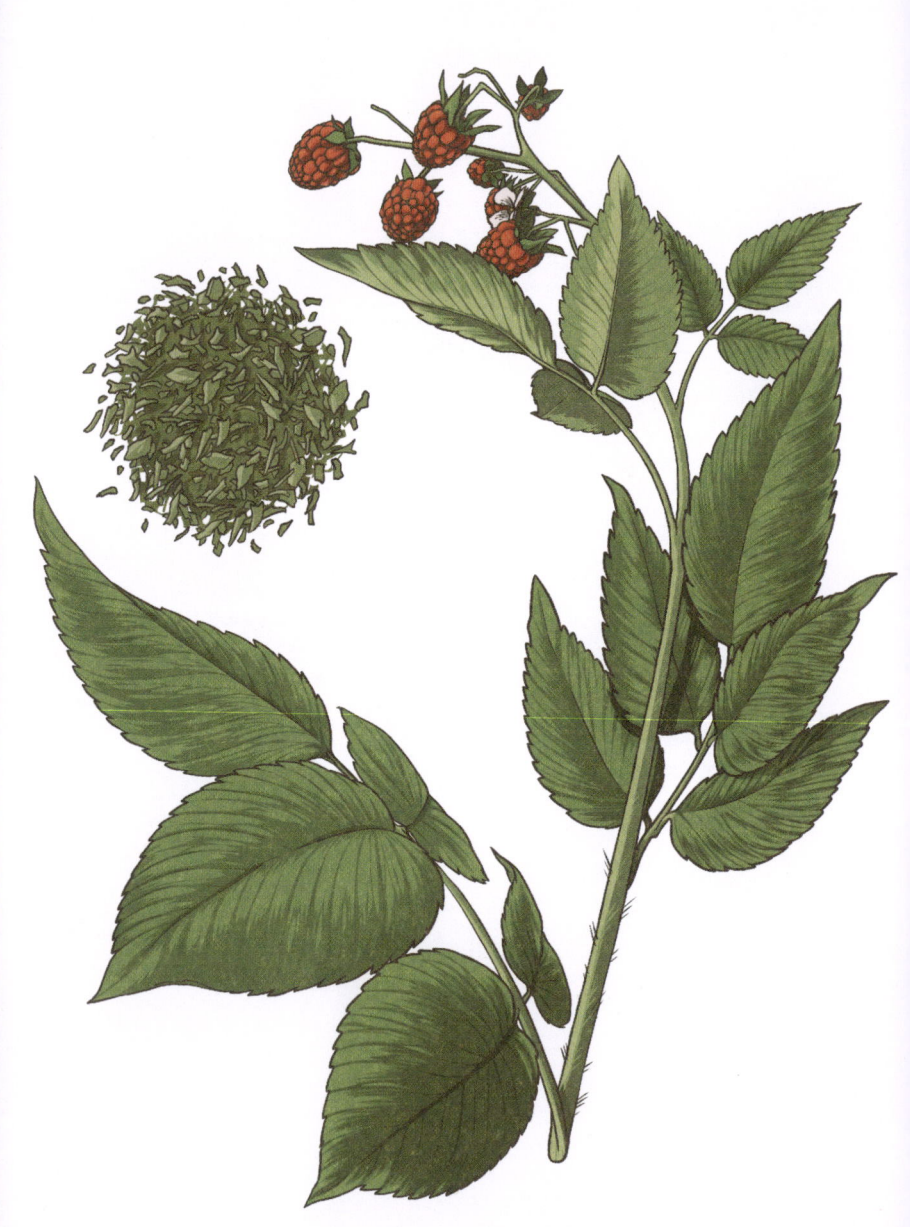

Raspberry

Rubus idaeus
Other name(s): red raspberry

Learning about red raspberry leaf as medicine proves amazing! Like blackberries, these summer berries offer more medicinal value than most realize. Red raspberry leaf contains iron, manganese, niacin, selenium, vitamins A and C, and calcium, plus tannins. Its primary use is as a uterine tonic to help with excessive menstrual bleeding and to tonify the uterus. In herbalism practice, it's used to prepare the uterus for labor and to reduce pain. M. Grieve recommends gargling with it for mouth or throat wounds, given its astringing properties. It also works as an external wash for sitz baths. It is best used as an infusion or tincture; the berries are edible!

PARTS USED: leaf and fruit

MEDICINAL USES: astringent, uterine tonic, antispasmodic, stimulant

SAFETY CONSIDERATIONS: Some practitioners advise against using raspberry leaf in the first trimester. Under knowledgeable practitioner care, moderate doses prove safe throughout pregnancy.

REMEDIES: Cramp Ease Tea, Herbal Iron Syrup, Iron Tea, Bone Strength Tea, Fertili-Tea, Mother's Nursing Blend, PMS Relief Tea, Raspberry Leaf Tea for Labor Support, After Birth Rebalance Tea, Beautiful Skin Herbal Facial Steam

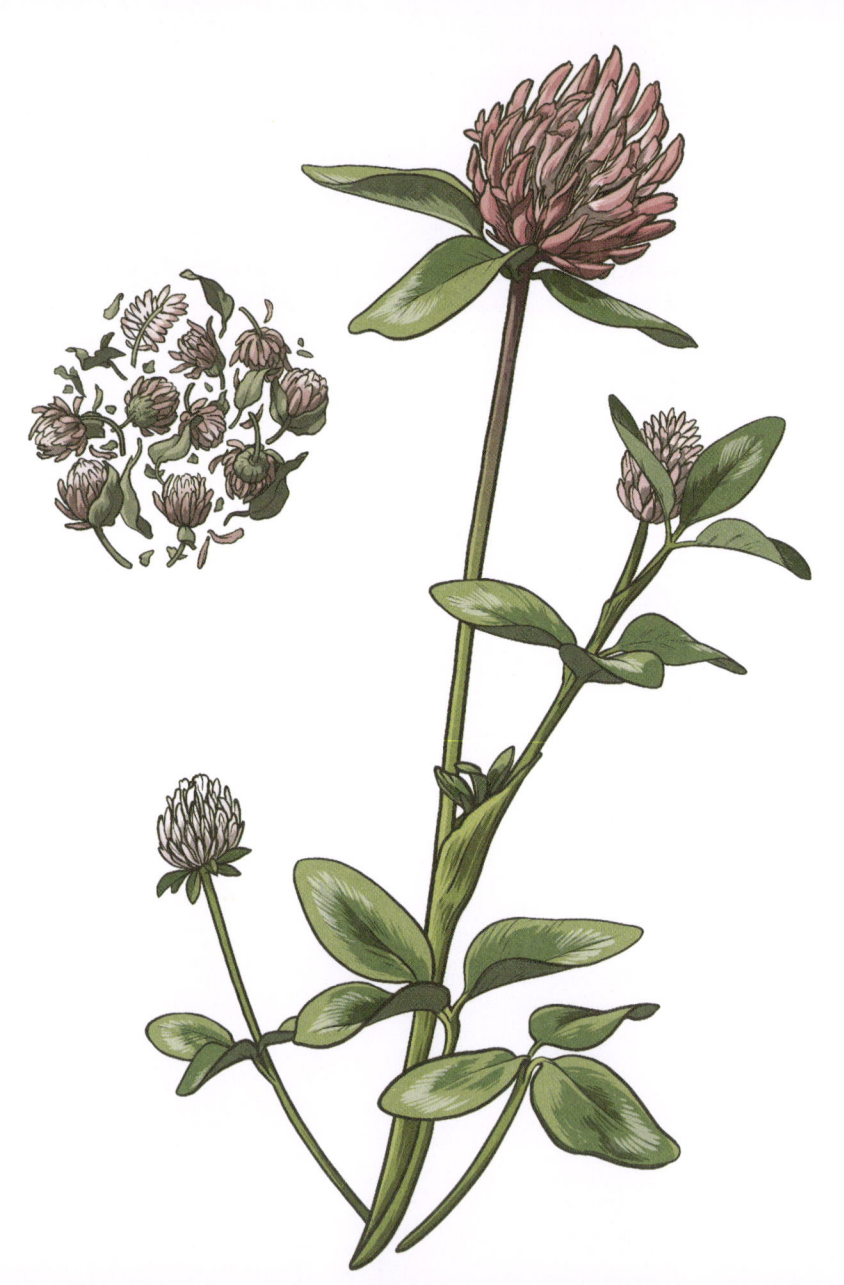

Red Clover

Trifolium pratense
Other name(s): none commonly used

Those yard weeds with the pinkish-purple blossoms are indeed medicine! Childhood memories include picking red clover from neighborhoods and sucking the blossoms (fairy food!). The red clover blossoms, or flowers, are sweet, cooling, and moistening, making them quite restorative and nourishing. The plant contains polysaccharides, calcium, chromium, magnesium, potassium, thiamin, and vitamin C. It also shows an affinity for blood purification and detoxification, helping skin issues like eczema or acne. With its estrogenic qualities, it can be helpful for women who are menstruating or in menopause and are experiencing sore throat, dry mouth, thirst, and hot flashes. It is best used as an infusion or tincture.

PARTS USED: flowers (also called buds or blossoms), leaf

MEDICINAL USES: diuretic, mild sedative, expectorant, blood detoxifier, estrogenic, antispasmodic

SAFETY CONSIDERATIONS: It is contraindicated during pregnancy (speculative). If used with estrogen replacement therapy it may cause excess estrogen.

REMEDIES: Gentle Liver Tonic Tea for Acne, Stop the Sweats Tincture, Mother's Nursing Blend, Daily Multivitamin Tea, Gentle Eczema Helper Tea, Gentle Liver Detox Formula, Long Life Oxymel

TIP: Only harvest from areas free of pesticides and pet traffic—roadside clover absorbs pollutants.

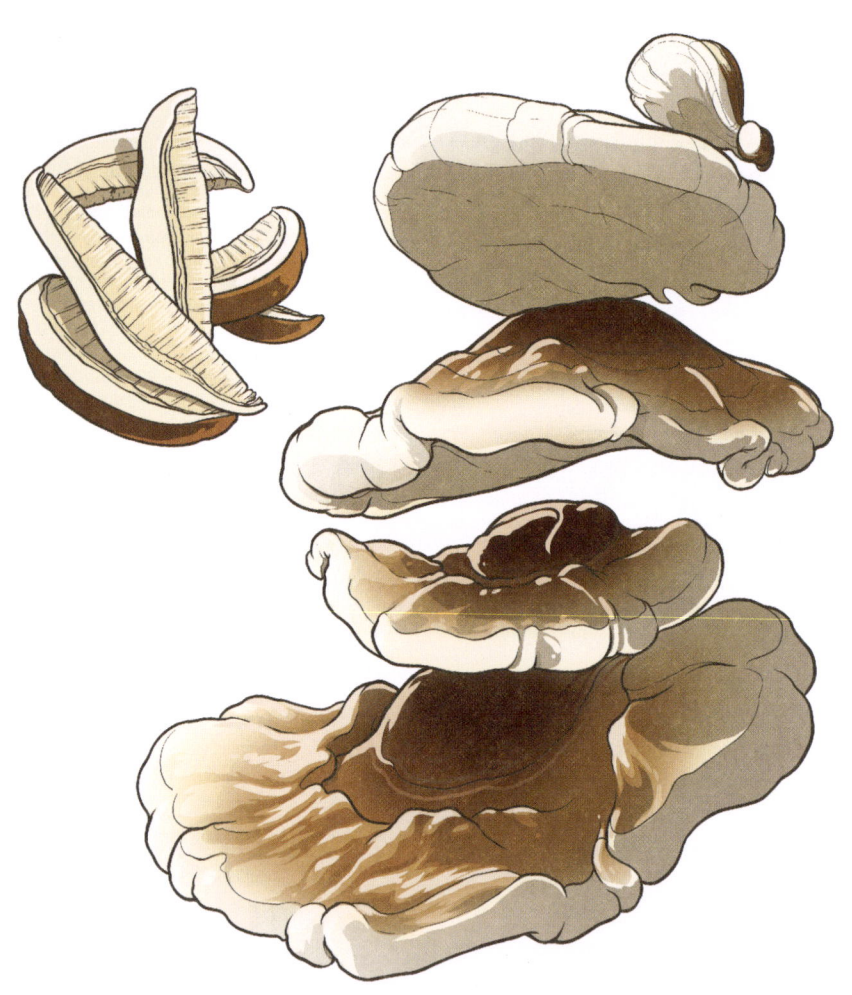

Reishi

Ganoderma lucidum
Other name(s): *ling zhi* (Chinese)

A powerful mushroom in Chinese medicine, reishi is tonifying to the whole system, especially the lungs, kidneys, and spleen. Daoists and Chinese medicine practitioners have revered it for centuries as a giver of life. Reishi is a tonic for Qi, which in Chinese medicine represents the vital energy that runs through our bodies—when someone has deficient Qi, they often experience chronic fatigue, frequent illness, loose stools, or chronic respiratory ailments such as asthma or shortness of breath. Reishi is best used as a decoction, powder, or tincture.

PARTS USED: whole mushroom

MEDICINAL USES: antiviral, antibacterial, anti-inflammatory, increases immunity, reduces cholesterol, regulates blood pressure

SAFETY CONSIDERATIONS: Qi tonics may cause bloating, headaches, or bowel irregularity if they're the wrong remedy for you or the dosage is too high.

REMEDIES: Immune Support Broth Blend, Root Beer Syrup

TIP: Start with small doses to assess your body's response— reishi can be quite powerful.

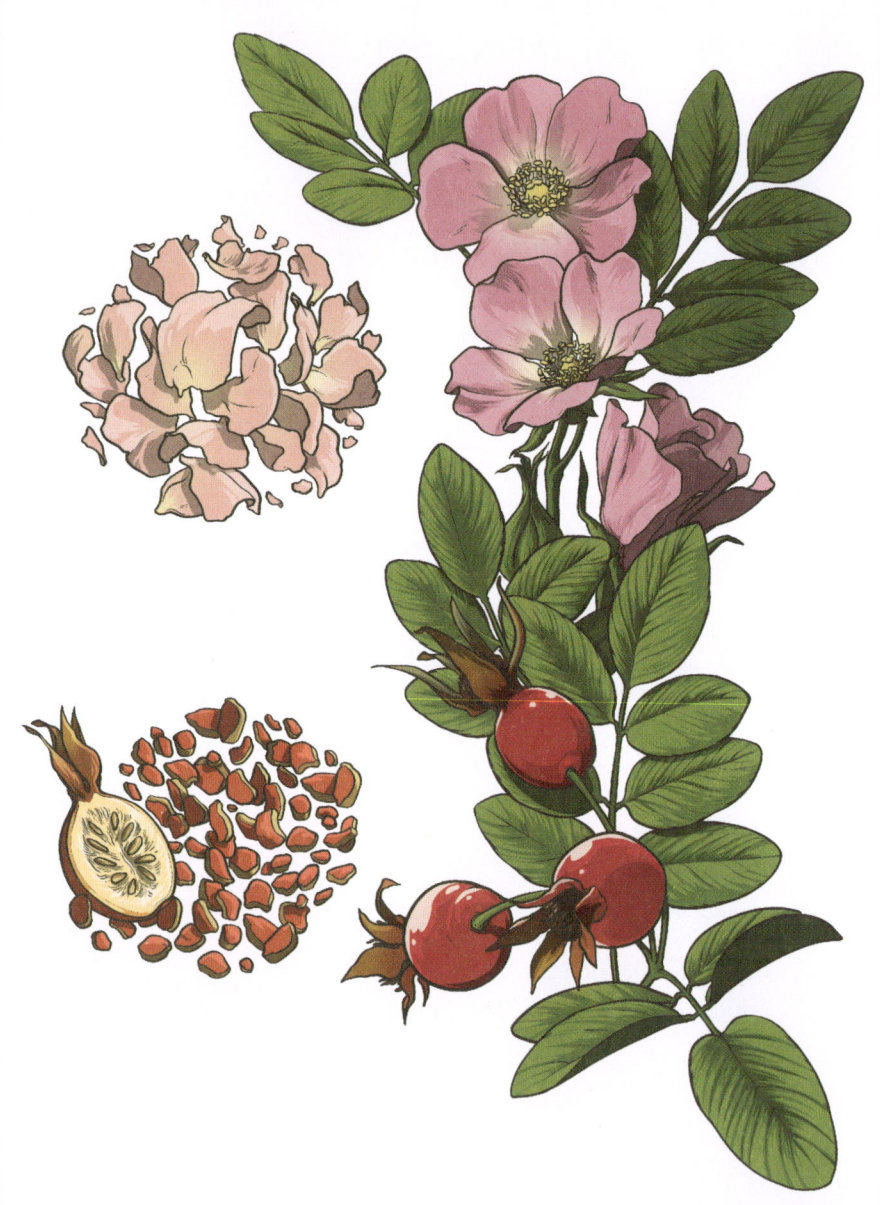

Rose

Rosa spp. including R. canina, R. rugosa,
R. multiflora and many others

Other name(s): dog rose (*rosa canina*), rugosa rose (*R. rugosa*),
multiflora rose, wild rose, baby rose (*R. multiflora*)

Roses are herbaceous shrubs that grow in all hemispheres. They're
generally aromatic, astringent, and sweet. In Chinese medicine, rose
addresses frustration or irritability. Roses also help late, heavy,
or painful periods. You've likely encountered rose in cosmetics,
skincare, or Middle Eastern cooking (rose water appears in several
recipes in this book!). Rose hips, the fruit that appears after summer flowers die, provide antioxidants, vitamin C, and quercetin,
which is astringent and heart supportive. Rose petals work best
in an infusion or tincture. Rose hips make excellent infusions,
tinctures, or syrups.

PARTS USED: petals, rose hips
(the dried fruit of roses)

MEDICINAL USES: anti-
inflammatory, antispasmodic,
moistening, wound healing,
mild antidepressant

SAFETY CONSIDERATIONS:
Many rose species exist—ensure
proper identification for inges-
tion when wildcrafting. Don't eat
rose hips raw.

REMEDIES: Acne Healing Vinegar,
Cramp Ease Tea, Uplifting
Nervous System Tonic, Soothing
Tummy Gummies, Herbal Bath
for Itchy Skin, Rose Cordial
for Rough Days, In-the-Mood
Damiana Cordial, Cold Kicker
Tea, Daily Multivitamin Tea, Long
Life Oxymel, Heart Healing Syrup

TIP: Beautiful ornamental
roses from the grocery stores
and florists typically aren't
the medicinal species to
use internally.

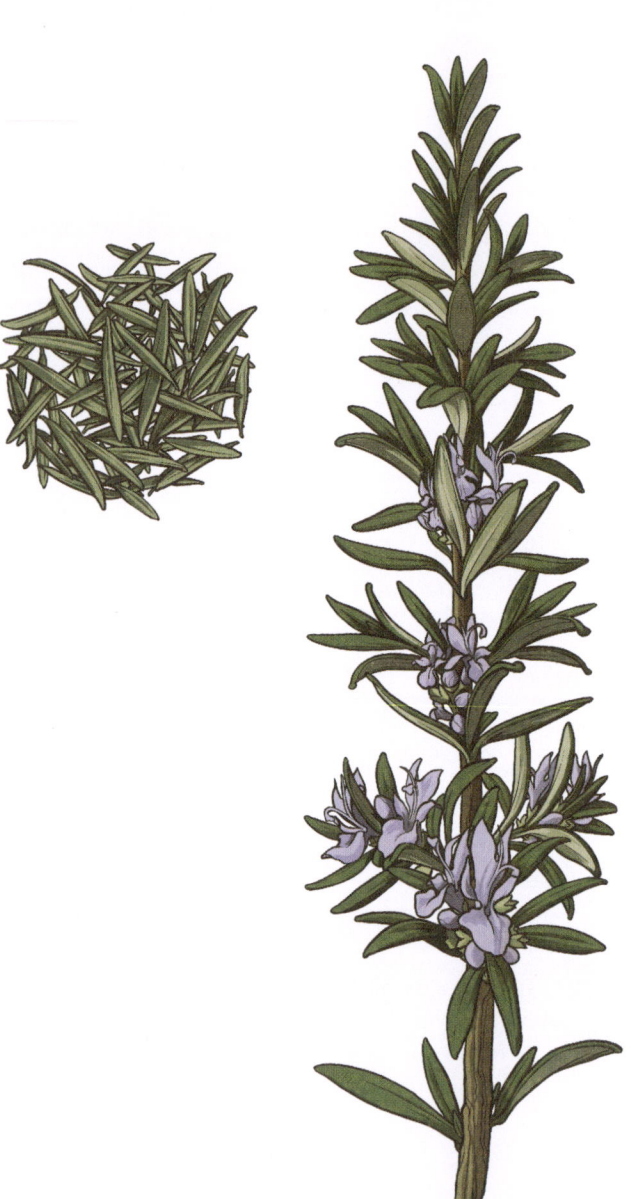

Rosemary

Rosmarinus officinalis
Other name(s): None commonly used

Rosemary brings an aromatic, warming, drying spiciness to kitchens and medicine cabinets alike! Used through the ages for memory enhancement, it carries a rich symbolic history in weddings, magic, and friendship. Its warming nature benefits circulation (helping cold hands and feet) and warms lungs to expel phlegm (or clear the sinuses during allergies or colds). Rosemary shows an affinity for the uterus, promoting healthy menstrual cycles or bringing on delayed periods (amenorrhea). It is an excellent treatment for headaches and works as a wash for various ailments and infections or in baths. It also serves as bug repellent. A few drops of this essential oil in a bath is divine! It is best used as an infusion, tincture, or essential oil.

PARTS USED: leaf

MEDICINAL USES: astringent, antibacterial, diaphoretic, diuretic, carminative, emmenagogue, antispasmodic, nervine, antioxidant

SAFETY CONSIDERATIONS: Use with caution in pregnancy due to its emmenagogue effect.

REMEDIES: Acne Healing Vinegar, Arthritis Alleviation Tea, The BEST Bug Spray, Warm Me Up Tea, Cold Kicking Vinegar, Stuffy Head Sinus Steam, Shiny Happy Healthy Hair Tea, Flaky Scalp Hair Rinse, Headache Relief Poultice, St John's Wort Sore Muscle Rub (essential oil), Post Partum Sitz Bath, Floral Herbal Toner

TIP: Fresh rosemary maintains potency for months when dried properly—hang bundles in dark, airy spaces.

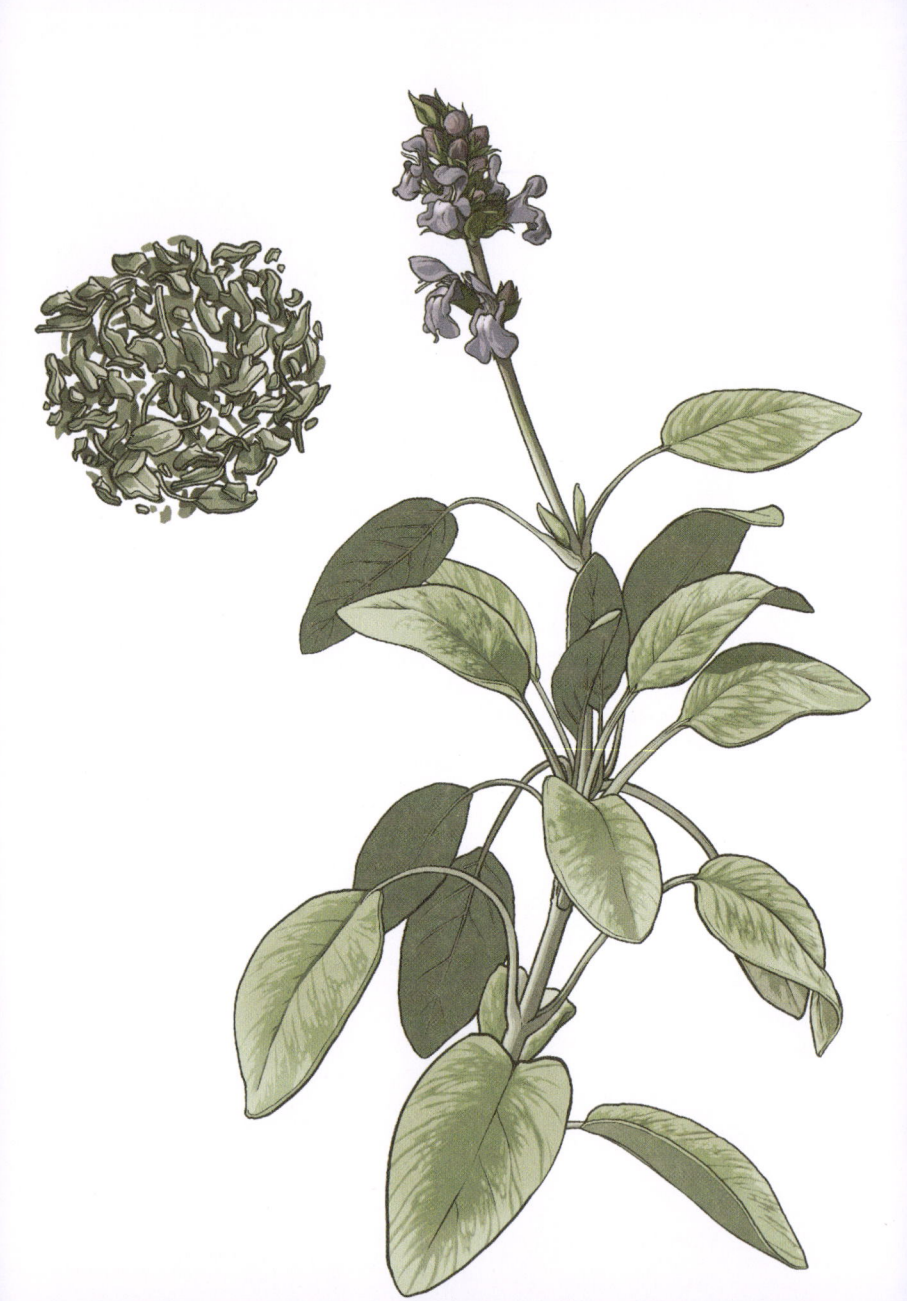

Sage

Salvia officinalis
Other name(s): garden sage, common sage

Sage can be used for more than Thanksgiving stuffing! This aromatic, bitter, cooling, and drying herb shows an affinity for stomach, intestine, uterus, lungs, brain, and nervous systems. It is high in zinc, vitamin A, magnesium, sodium, and thiamine. It works beautifully as a reproductive tonic, helping with labor and estrogen imbalances that cause night sweats and hot flashes. It also tonifies the nervous system while addressing excessive sweating. For throat infections, gargle or drink as a tea for its antiseptic and wound-healing properties. It is best used as an infusion or tincture (or just add to your cooking!).

PART USED: leaf

MEDICINAL USES: astringent, antibacterial, carminative, uterine stimulant

SAFETY CONSIDERATIONS: It is contraindicated during pregnancy due to its emmenagogue effects. It may reduce milk flow.

REMEDIES: Cool Me Down Hot Flash Tincture, Stop the Sweats Tincture, Cold Kicking Vinegar (optional addition), Stuffy Head Sinus Steam

TIP: This is garden sage. White sage, popular for smudging, is entirely different—a sacred Native American plant best reserved for those with ancestral heritage connections.

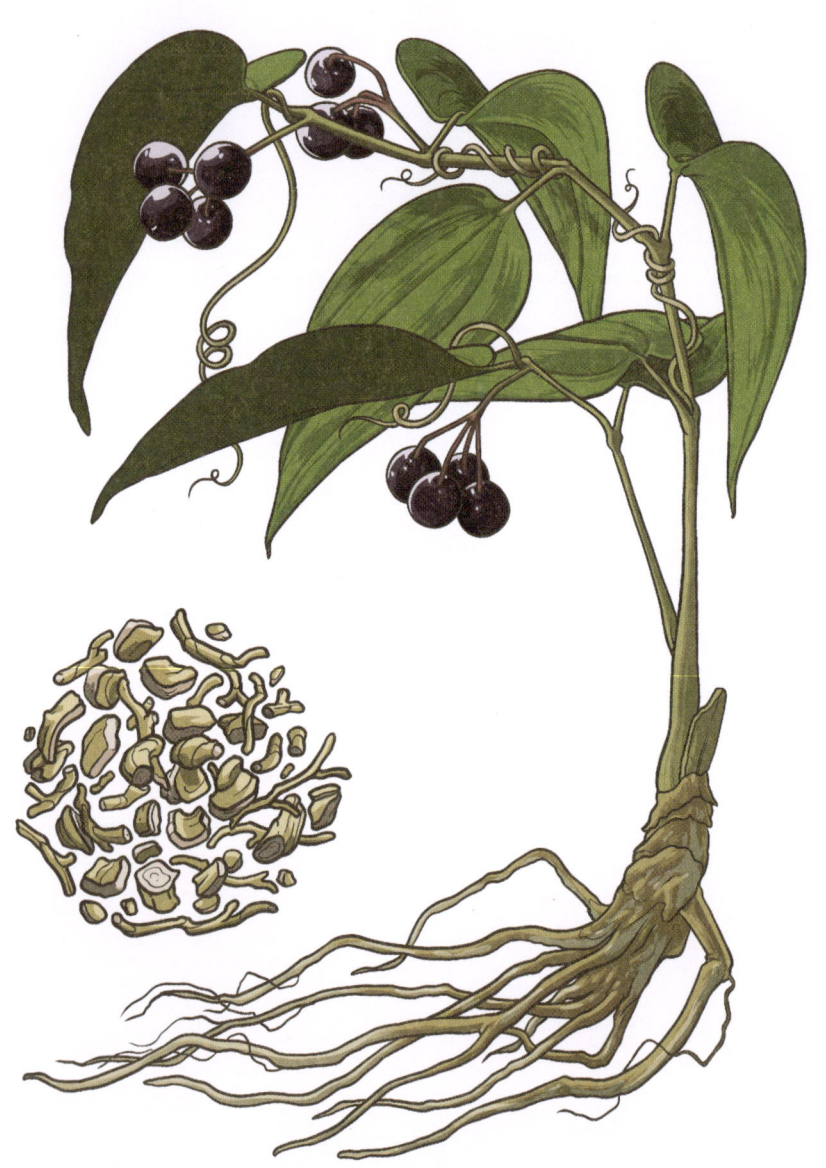

Sarsaparilla

Smilax spp.
Other name(s): None commonly used

Sarsaparilla comes from perennial vines growing in Central and South America—you know it best as root beer flavoring! This slightly drying, sweet, and slightly mucilaginous root has historical use as a blood and lymph tonic. It is excellent for treating hormonal imbalances and skin conditions such as psoriasis. It's high in selenium, iron, silicon, and zinc. This plant is valued as an alternative herb, meaning it helps the body process nutrition and repair bodily tissue and changes, like an adaptogen. It "alters" the body's function beneficially. It can also aid in digestion. It is best used as a decoction, long infusion, or tincture.

PARTS USED: root

MEDICINAL USES: diuretic, diaphoretic, anti-inflammatory, antibacterial

SAFETY CONSIDERATIONS: Dr. Tilgner notes contraindication during pregnancy, though literature elsewhere doesn't specify why.

REMEDIES: Women's Rooted Tea, Root Beer Syrup, Psoriasis Relief Tea

TIP: Different species of this plant can vary significantly in taste. If you come across one that isn't sweet enough to your liking, try another source—products from different regions (for example, one from South America and another from elsewhere) can have noticeably different flavor profiles.

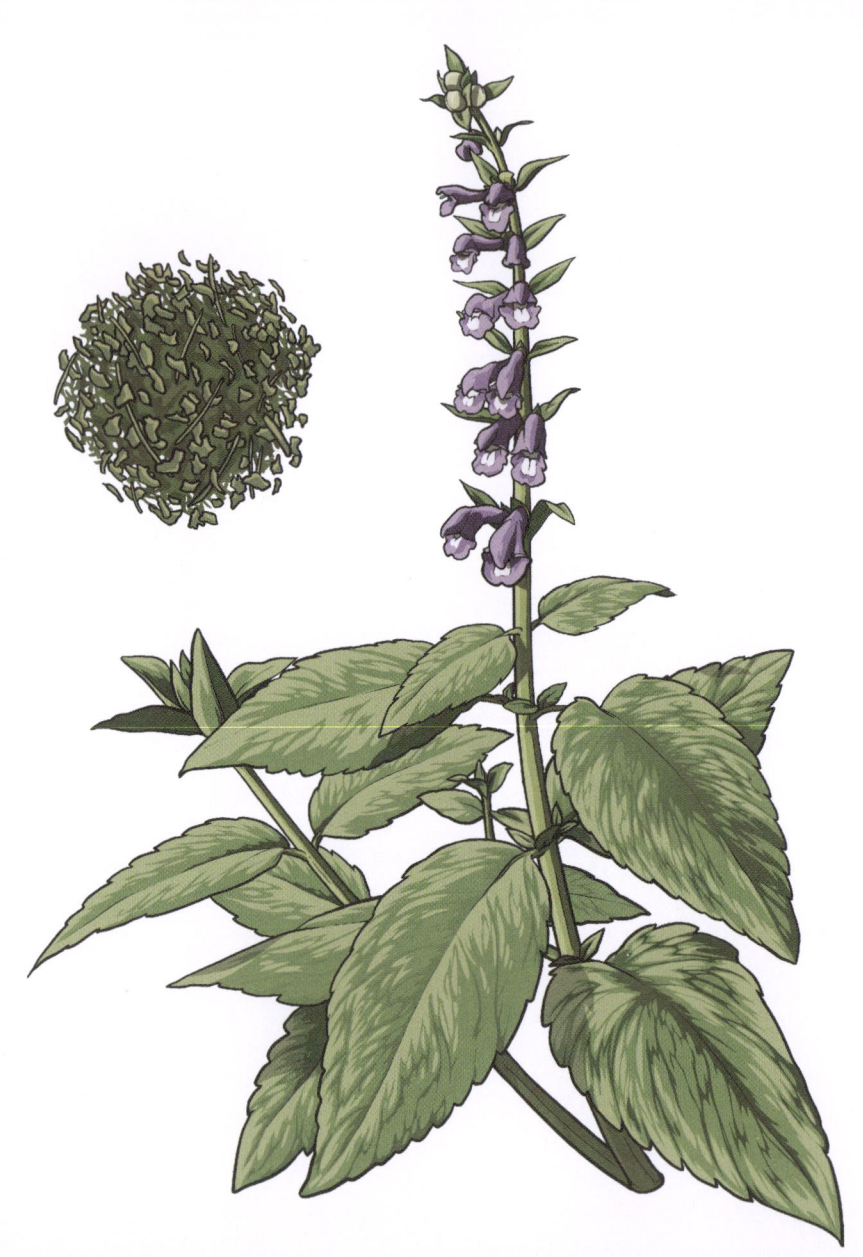

Skullcap

Scutellaria lateriflora
Other name(s): American skullcap, scullcap,
blue scullcap, mad-dog weed

Skullcap is a bitter, cooling, mint-family plant with affinity for the heart, nerves, liver, and kidneys. It's high in minerals, including zinc. Once known as "mad-dog weed" for historically helping to treat canine rabies, it's used chiefly in humans for nervousness, restlessness, and pain. The combination of nervous system calming, antibacterial properties, and antispasmodic action makes it perfect for stress-related illness and tension. Its cousin, Baikal skullcap root (*huang qin*), serves entirely different purposes in Chinese medicine—much more bitter and draining. American skull-cap proves more tonifying and restorative and also helps a nervous stomach. It is best used as an infusion or tincture.

PARTS USED: aerial parts

MEDICINAL USES: nervine, sedative, anti-inflammatory, antispasmodic, hypotensive, antibacterial

SAFETY CONSIDERATIONS: none noted

REMEDIES: Get to Sleep Tea, Pain Relieving Tea, Stress Relief Tea

TIP: Try this herb on its own as a tea or tincture to support sleep, ease anxiety, or relieve general tension.

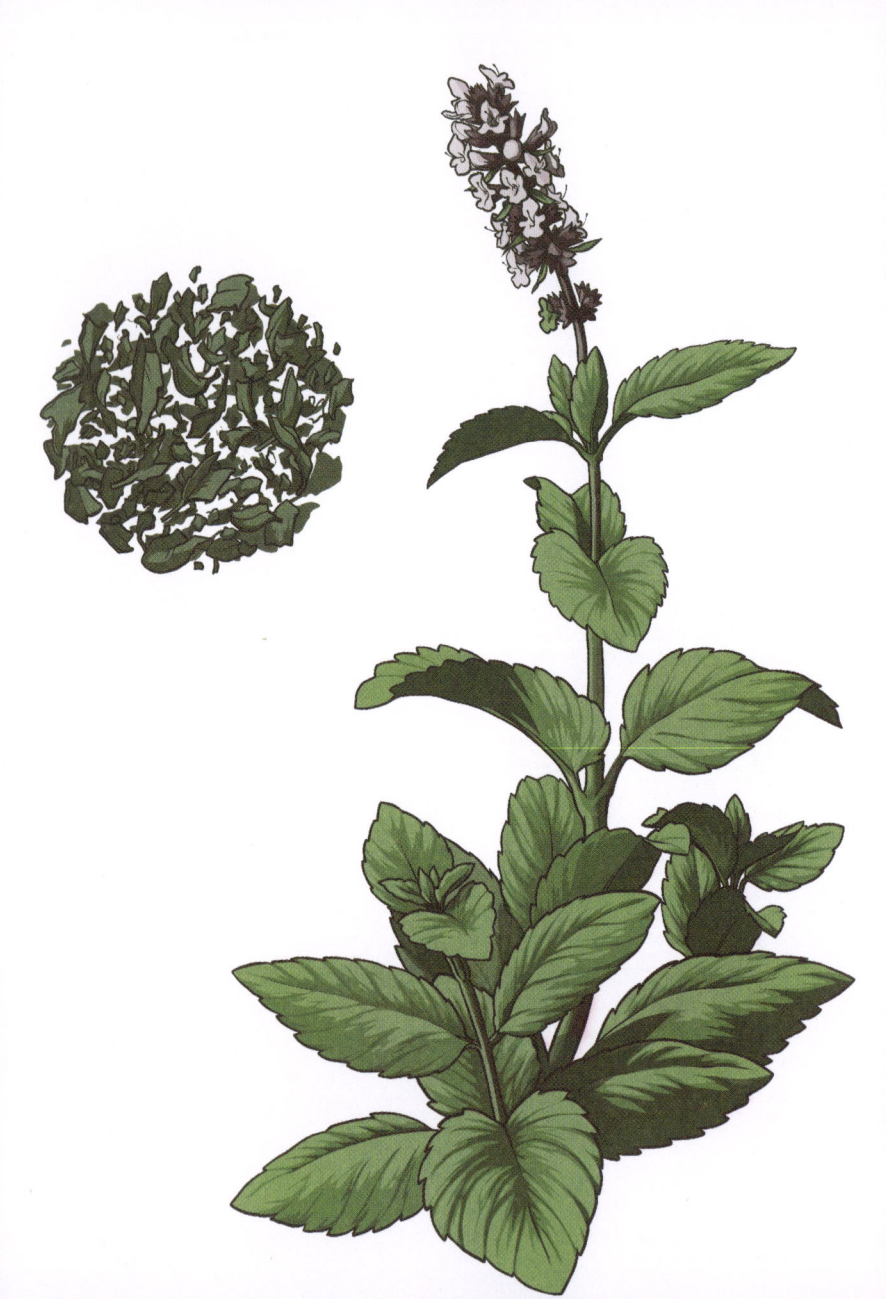

Spearmint

Mentha spicata
Other name(s): none commonly used

Many mints are full of vitamins and minerals—spearmint is no exception. Sweet, cooling, and aromatic, it is simultaneously relaxing and stimulating while restoring lungs, stomach, bladder, and kidneys. It contains iron, sodium, silicon, copper, and vitamins A and C. In upper respiratory infections it relieves sore throat, fever, and cough. It can settle the stomach or be combined with peppermint for soothing a tummy or for a midday wake-up instead of coffee. It can aid with urinary tract inflammation (combine with mullein, marshmallow, and plantain for a soothing diuretic effect). It is best used as an infusion or tincture.

PARTS USED: leaf, flower

MEDICINAL USES: antipyretic (can help reduce fevers), digestive aid, sedative, anti-inflammatory, diuretic, antispasmodic

SAFETY CONSIDERATIONS: None available at this time

REMEDIES: Gentle Liver Tonic Tea for Acne, Iron Tea (optional addition), Arthritis Alleviation Tea (optional addition), Bye-Bye Bloat Tea, Clear the Fog Tea, Cool Down and Rehydrate Tea, Rehydrating Tea for the Runs, Root Beer Syrup, Women's Rooted Tea, Cool Me Down Hot Flash Tincture (optional addition, Fertili-Tea, Lymph Mover Tea (optional addition), soothing Tea for Nausea, PMS Relief Tea

TIP: If spearmint makes you think of toothpaste, give it a second chance! The fresh plant has a mild, natural sweetness that may surprise you.

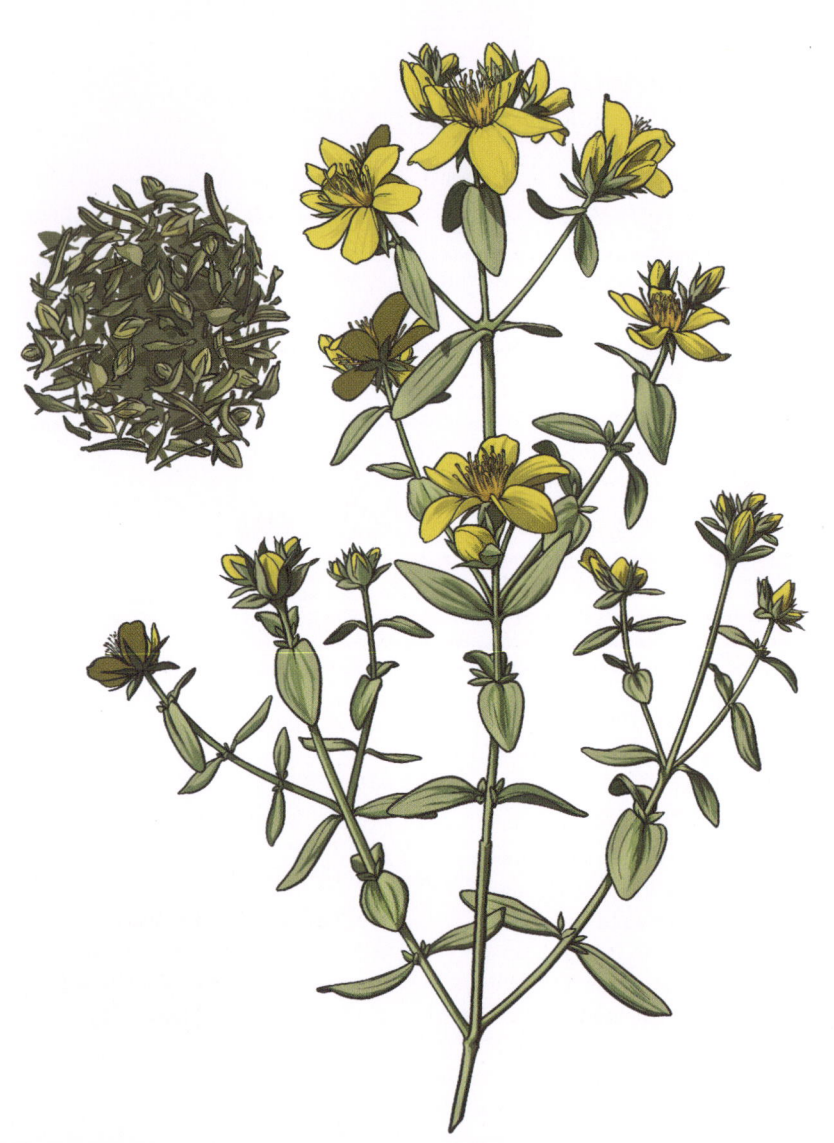

48

St. John's Wort

Hypericum perforatum
Other name(s): St. Joan's wort, witches herb, touch-and-heal

St. John's wort offers slightly bitter, astringent, and mild warming qualities with bright yellow flowers that reach full bloom in July. It is known for helping depression, anxiety, and mood disorders. It is best to use it fresh for medicine-making—gently squeeze the unopened buds to see the red liquid emerge (the good stuff!), creating a beautiful red oil. It is an excellent nervine for nerve pain and shingles. It can help with winter depression after sunless periods, depression with irritability, frustration, or unresolved anger. It is great for perimenopause or menopause. St. John's wort works low and slow—usually taking several diligent weeks for results. It is best used as an infusion, tincture of the fresh plant, or topically (with the oil of the fresh plant).

PARTS USED: flowering tops—mix of almost-opened buds, full flowers, and a little stem (mostly buds)

MEDICINAL USES: antiviral, anti-inflammatory, antibacterial, wound-healing, nervine, sedative, antidepressant

SAFETY CONSIDERATIONS: It is contraindicated during pregnancy due to emmenagogue effects. It could cause photosensitivity in fair-skinned people. It may inhibit serotonin uptake—use cautiously with antidepressants to avoid reducing medication effectiveness.

St. John's wort is the most studied herb for contraindications. These contraindications apply to internal use; topical use for pain remains safe.

REMEDIES: Kick That Cold Sore Tea, St. John's Wort Tincture, St. John's Wort Oil and St. John's Wort Sore Muscle Rub

TIP: This herb can increase irritability in some people—try lower doses (a few drops daily instead of the standard 2 dropperfuls 2 to 3 times daily) or capsules.

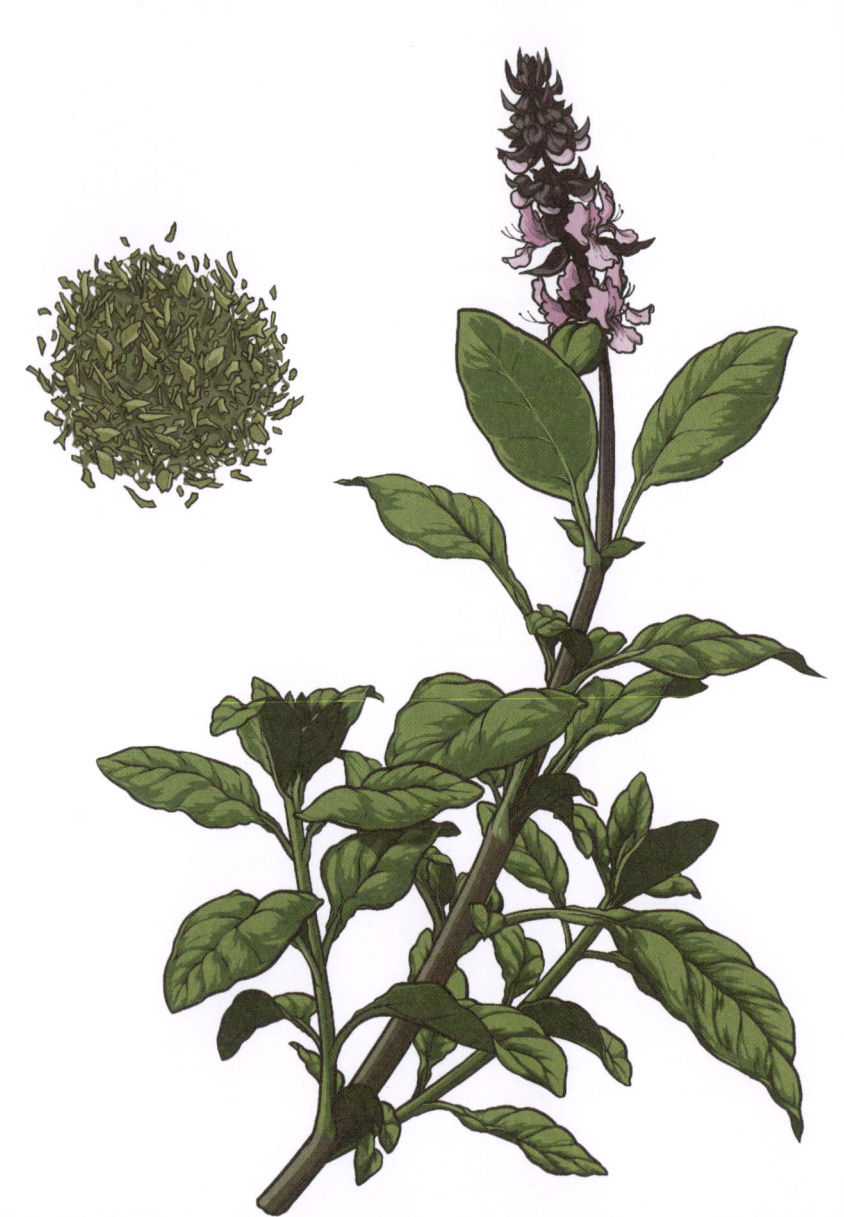

49

Tulsi

Ocimum sanctum
Other name(s): holy basil, *vishnupriya* ("The beloved one of Vishnu")

Tulsi, or holy basil, is an Ayurvedic dark-green leafy herb—hot, pungent, bitter, and considered one of India's three most sacred herbs, along with soma and lotus. I discovered love at first taste in K. P. Khalsa's class featuring a tulsi-rose tea—so pleasant, delicious, and calming (I still use it today). A member of the basil genus (*Ocimum*), it is unlike American basil—much spicier, more fragrant, and bitter. Tasting it brings immediate warmth—a diaphoretic help with colds and flu, and useful for fevers. It has proved helpful as an antidepressant (especially with rose), a mild stimulant (with peppermint or spearmint), a relaxant, and a pain reliever. K. P. used it for diabetes, cardiovascular health, hypertension, and blood sugar support. It is best used as an infusion or tincture.

PARTS USED: leaf

MEDICINAL USES: diaphoretic, stimulant, antidepressant, antioxidant, carminative, digestive aid, antispasmodic

SAFETY CONSIDERATIONS: No known safety considerations at this time

REMEDIES: Dry Those Drips Tea, Clear the Fog Tea, Warm Me Up Tea, Let the Sun In Tea

TIP: Multiple tulsi varieties exist with different flavor profiles—*Vana*, *Rama*, and *Krishna* are most common. Some taste pepperier, others lemonier. Try blends of all three!

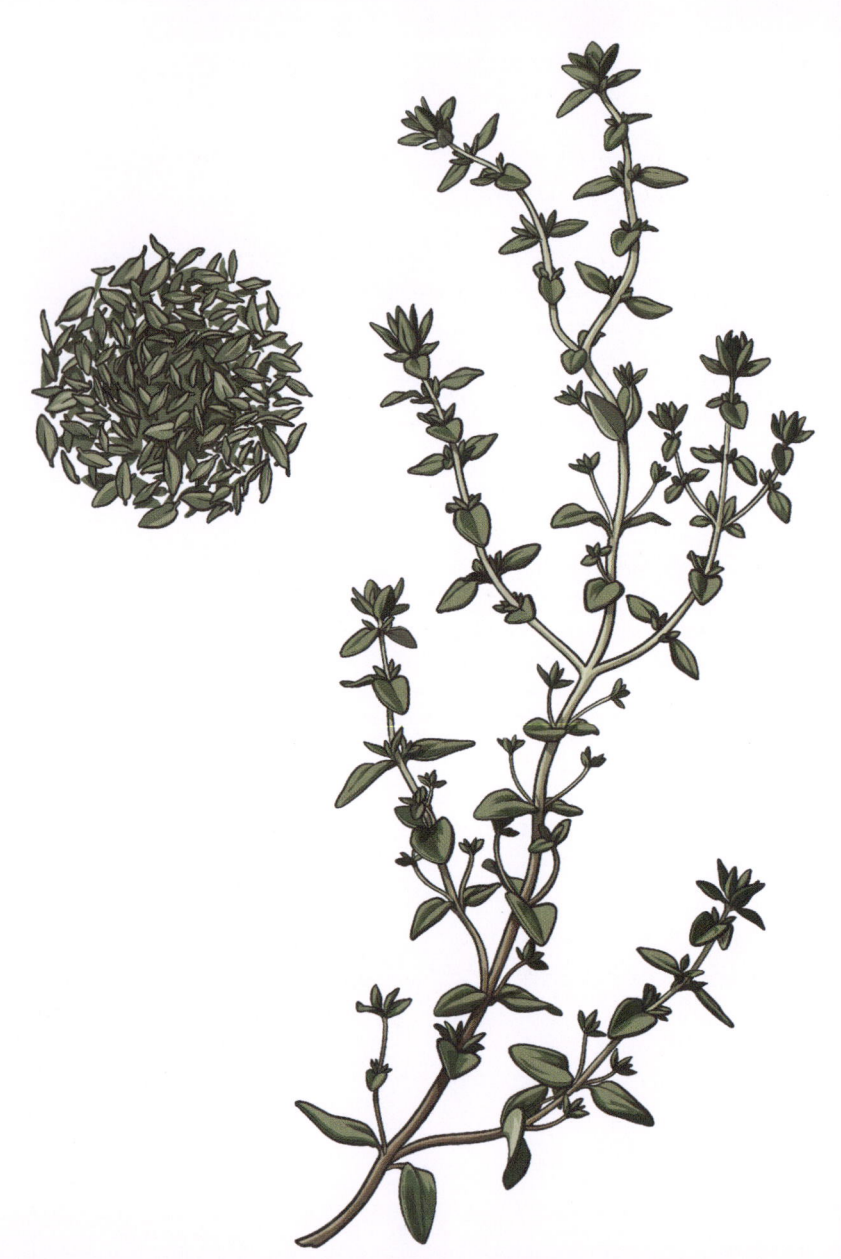

50

Thyme

Thymus vulgaris
Other name(s): garden thyme

Thyme is an aromatic, warming, pungent, and drying plant with an affinity for the lungs, stomach, intestines, and nerves. Aside from being a tasty common kitchen herb, thyme is used most for its warming components for the lungs, supporting bronchial conditions and the onset of colds and flu with painful, congested sinuses. It's also helpful for digestive issues accompanying colds, like watery or loose stools, digestive pain, and low appetite (may also help certain types of intestinal parasites). Some common kitchen herbs—rosemary, sage, marjoram, thyme—contain potent essential oils, making them strong bacteria killers (explaining their historical use as cooking spices when food spoilage threatened). Thyme tonifies and strengthens weak, nervous immune systems. It is best used as an infusion, tincture, or essential oil.

PARTS USED: leaves primarily, flowers

MEDICINAL USES: expectorant, antispasmodic, antioxidant, antibacterial, antifungal, diuretic

SAFETY CONSIDERATIONS: Be careful not to overuse this plant, as high doses might cause digestive upset.

REMEDIES: Cold Kicking Vinegar, Stuffy Head Sinus Steam, Flaky Scalp Hair Rinse

TIP: A small pot of thyme on the porch is a lovely addition to any home. If you buy a packet from the store for cooking and don't use it all, consider repurposing the leftovers as tea or in any of the recipes in this book. No herb should go to waste!

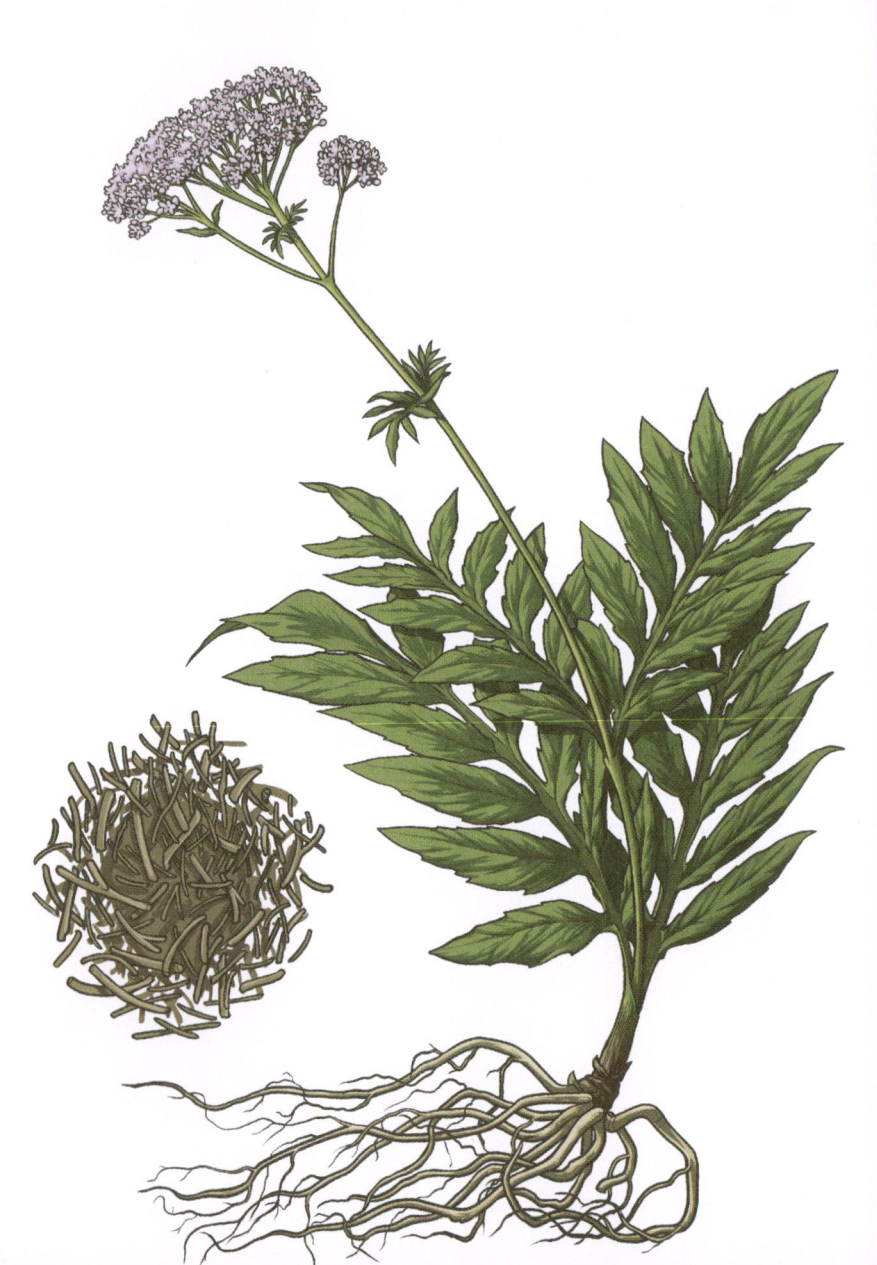

51

Valerian

Valeriana officinalis
Other name(s): none commonly used

Valerian root brings aromatic, sweet yet spicy, slightly warming
qualities, most notably sedating to help sleep. Plants grow tall
with tiny, starlike white flowers emitting a seductive scent. Some
dislike the valerian root's smell, but many find it almost seductive,
drawing them into dreamlike sleepy states (perfect for falling asleep
troubles!). My first encounter with its flowers led to trancelike
napping after endless inhalation. Its root helps all spasmodic
conditions—coughs, muscle spasms, pain, anxiety with agitation,
and restlessness. It is best used as an infusion or tincture.

PARTS USED: root

MEDICINAL USES: sedative,
nervine, antispasmodic, diuretic,
hypotensive, diaphoretic

SAFETY CONSIDERATIONS:
Be cautious when combining
valerian with sleep aids such
as barbiturates, as it enhances
their effects.

REMEDIES: Get to Sleep Tea,
Cough Syrup (optional for
spasmodic cough)

TIP: Valerian isn't a long-term
insomnia solution. Effects
diminish with continuous use.
Take breaks, use other herbs,
and work with professionals to
address underlying sleep issues.

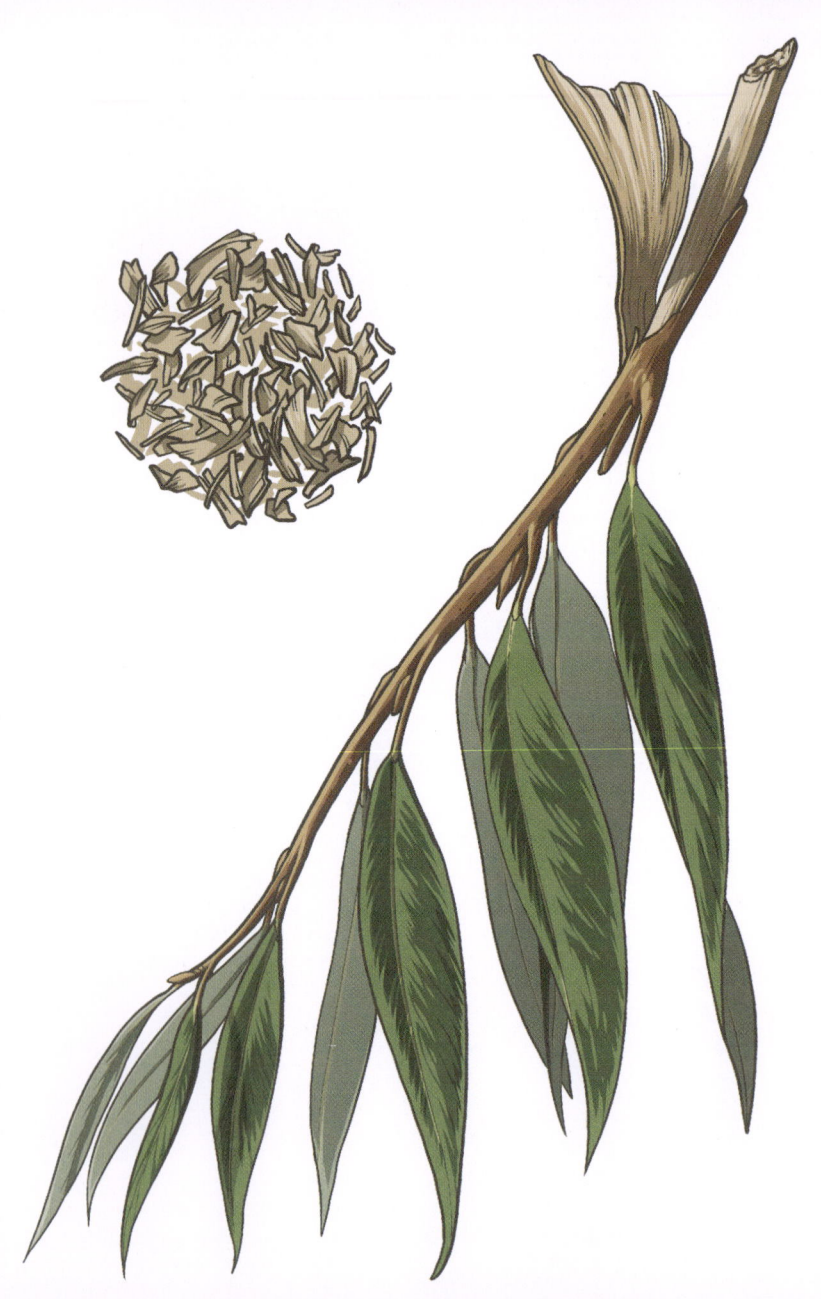

Willow Bark

Salix spp.
Other name(s): white willow bark, sallow tree

Willow trees grow whimsically by riverbanks—sitting under their weeping branches while watching leaves dance brings spring and summer joy. The bark provides medicine—astringent, bitter, cooling, drying—mostly for pain relief. It can be used for headaches, fever, and various body aches. Willow bark's salicylic acid content historically proved harsh on stomachs, leading Felix Hoffmann at Friedrich Bayer and Company to seek solutions in the late 1800s. He discovered the acetyl ester component of salicylic acid, leading Bayer to market aspirin in 1899. It is best used as a decoction or tincture.

PARTS USED: bark

MEDICINAL USES: anti-inflammatory, astringent, analgesic, antiseptic

SAFETY CONSIDERATIONS: It is contraindicated with anticoagulants as it is a blood-mover.

REMEDIES: Willow Bark Tincture for Head Pain, Beautiful Skin Herbal Facial Steam

TIP: Willow bark in teas tastes very bitter and may upset stomachs—a tincture often proves gentler while maintaining effectiveness.

NOTE: There may be some dispute if Hoffmann was the original discoverer of this compound, as written in this article in PubMed: Sneader W. "The Discovery of Aspirin: A Reappraisal."

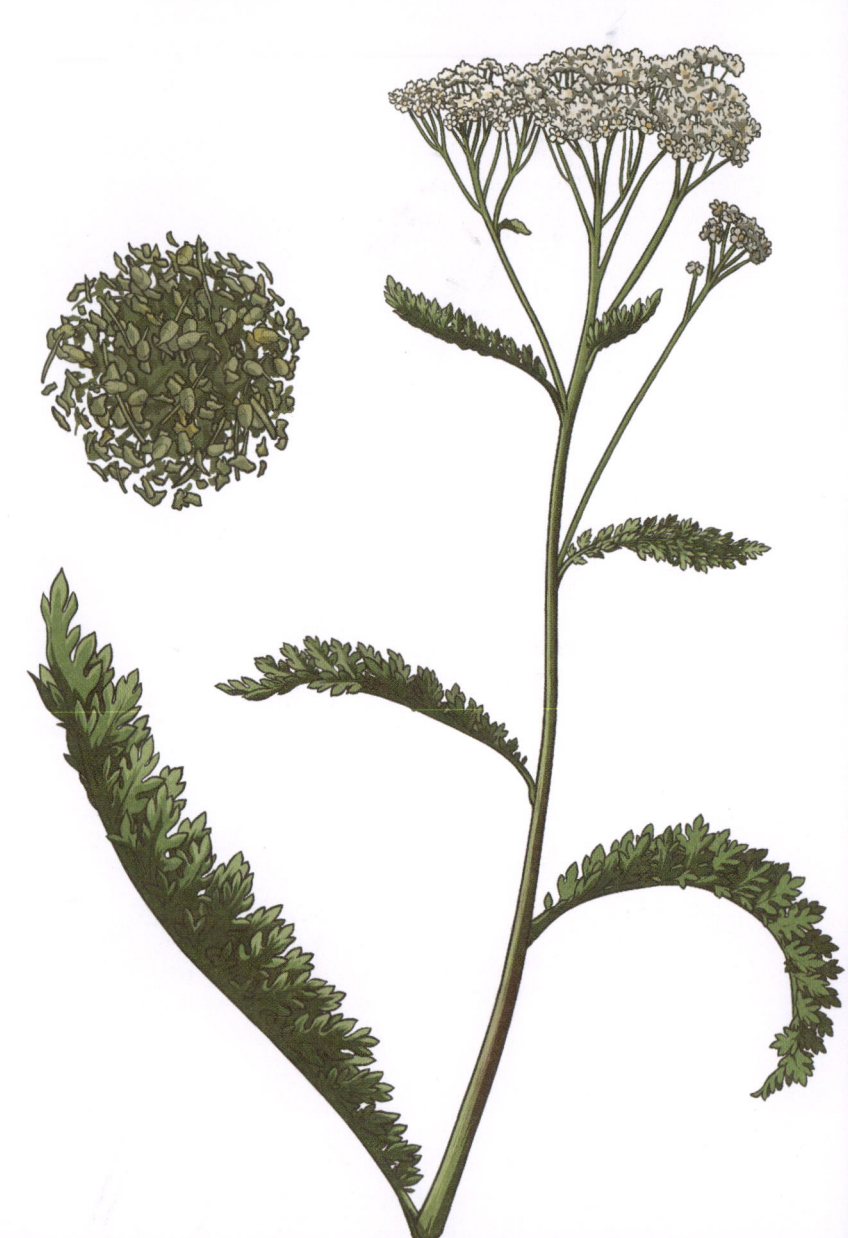

Yarrow

Achillea millefolium

Other name(s): milfoil, thousand weed, nosebleed, devil's nettle

Yarrow blooms beautifully in summer with white, lilac, or pink flowers resembling hundreds of flattened daisies in umbrella-like tops. Bitter, aromatic, astringent, cooling, and drying with an affinity for many body systems, it is commonly used as diaphoretic venting fevers, especially in the upper body. Its Latin name *Achillea* reflects its wound-healing abilities, touted by Achilles to staunch the bleeding wounds of his soldiers. Its species name *millefolium,* refers to the many segments of its foliage—the leaves are wispy and silky. It has been used magically to "ward off the Evil One" and for protection talismans. It is an excellent aid for circulation, warming, and regulating menstrual cycles (especially with strong PMS). It can be used as a digestive bitter tonic and stimulator and for inflammation and tissue healing. Mix with ginger and cinnamon to use at the onset of a cold (or when feeling cold). It is best used as an infusion or tincture.

PARTS USED: flowers and leaves

MEDICINAL USES: diaphoretic, astringent, antiseptic, antifungal, anti-inflammatory, anticoagulant, wound healing

SAFETY CONSIDERATIONS: It is contraindicated during pregnancy due to its emmenagogue effects.

REMEDIES: Stuffy Head Sinus Steam, Fever Diminish Tea, Sore Muscle Compress

TIP: Many yarrow colors exist, even dark magenta! White yarrow predominates in clinical use.

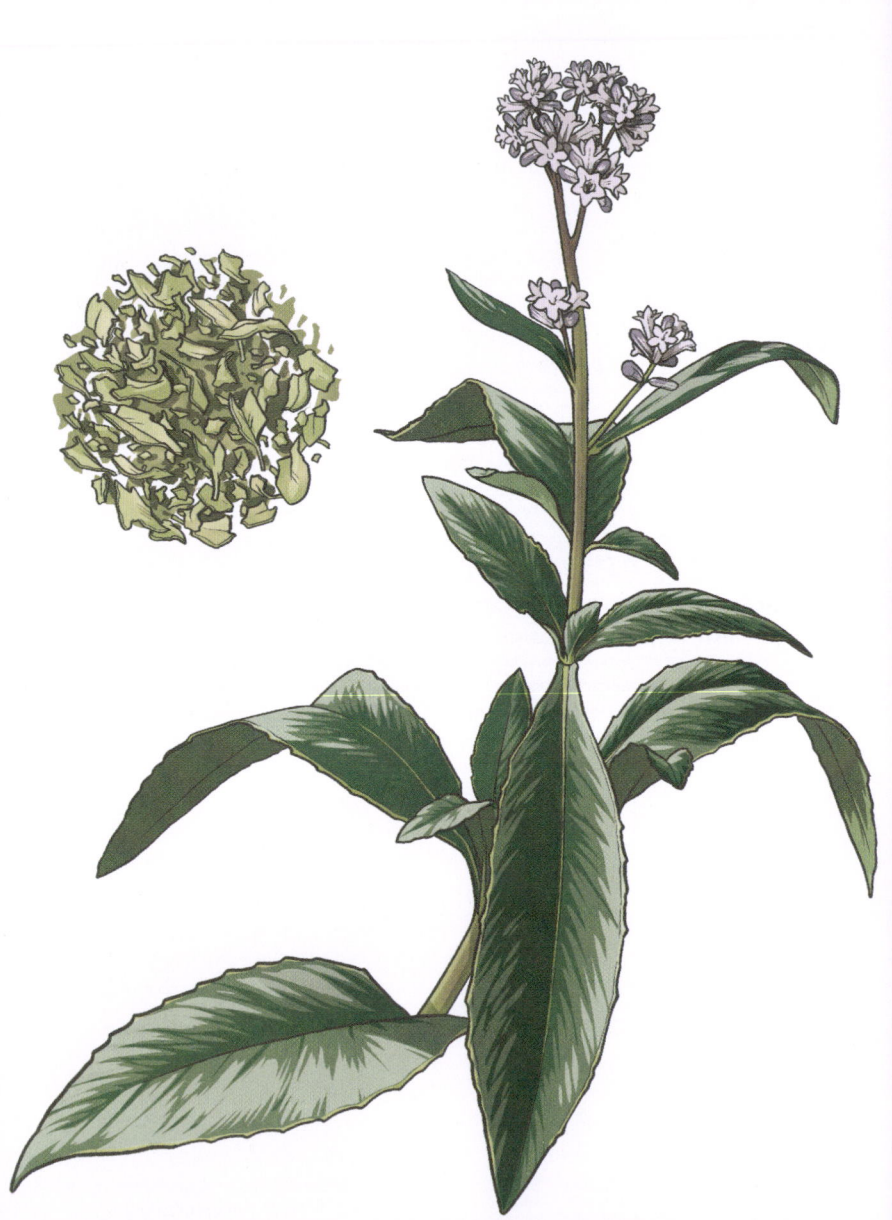

Yerba Santa

Eriodictyon californicum
Other name(s): mountain balm, bear plant, holy herb

Yerba santa brings very warming, aromatic, sweet, slightly bitter qualities with an affinity for lungs, stomach, and head (especially sinuses). This low desert shrub from the Southwest mountains and Northern Mexico contains iron, magnesium, niacin, phosphorus, selenium, and vitamins A and C. It is most useful for lung conditions with damp phlegm, wheezing, and coughing with sinus congestion. It also addresses similar allergy presentations. As a carminative, it helps a cold, gassy stomach. It is best used as an infusion or tincture.

PARTS USED: leaves

MEDICINAL USES: expectorant, carminative, bronchodilator

SAFETY CONSIDERATIONS: No known safety considerations at this time

REMEDIES: Dry Those Drips Tea

TIP: Add this herb to any blend targeting congestion. If it causes dryness, consider removing it from the formula or balancing it with marshmallow root or another mucilaginous herb to help retain moisture in the body.

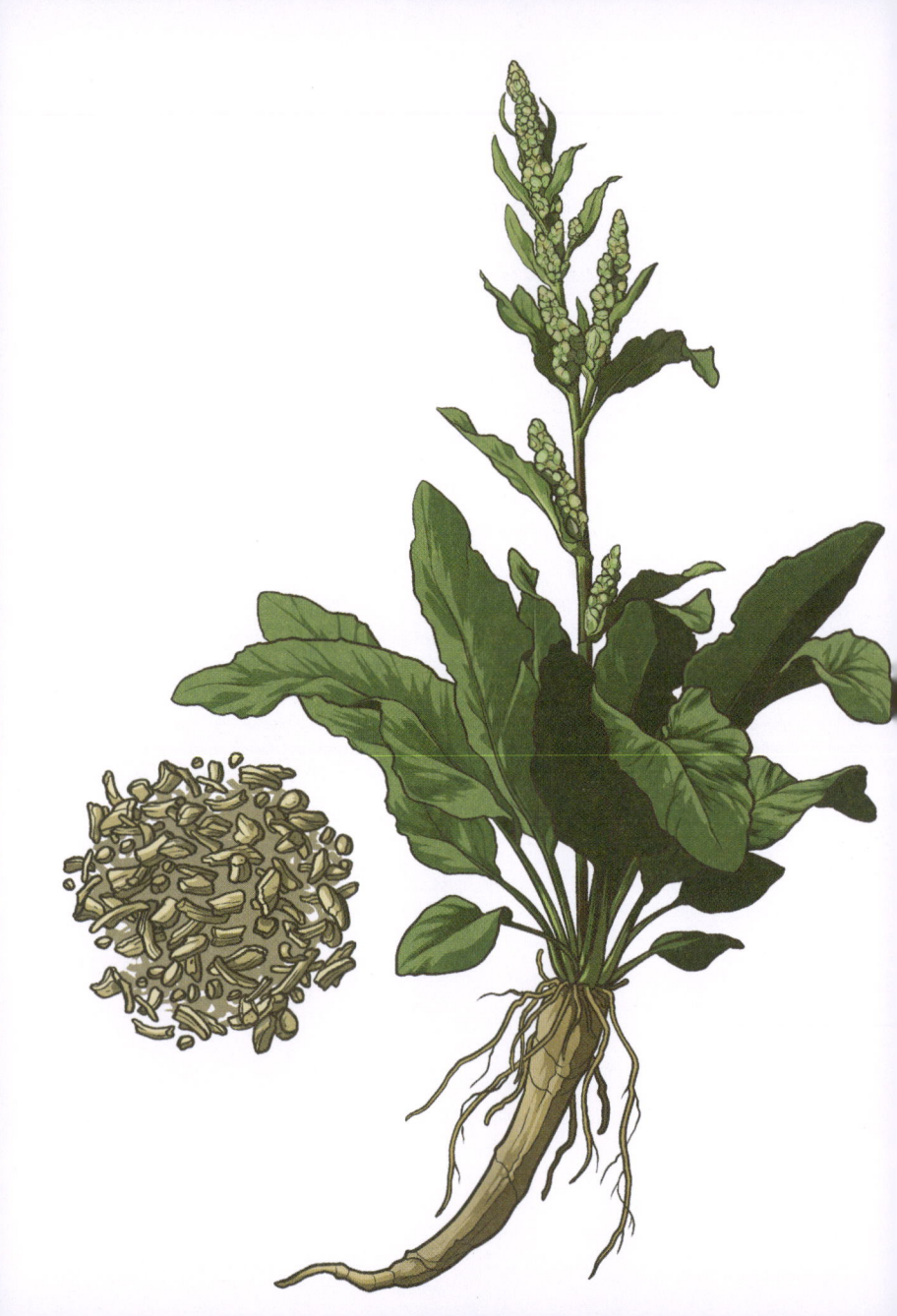

Yellow Dock

Rumex crispus, R. obtusifolius
Other name(s): curled dock, narrow-leaf dock (*R. crispus*),
broad-leafed dock (*R. obtusifolius*)

Yellow dock provides astringent, bitter, cooling properties with affinity for lymph, intestines, skin, and blood. *R. crispus* commonly appears in medicine, but broad-leafed dock (*R. obtusifolius*) grows abundantly in Seattle—they're nearly identical medicinally. The root serves as primary medicine, though young leaves can be collected and eaten (they require blanching then boiling due to oxalate content). Yellow dock's antimicrobial and astringent properties benefit skin conditions, digestive disorders with loose bowels or constipation, and bleeding hemorrhoids. Its decent iron content makes it useful for anemia recipes, and it also provides liver and gallbladder tonic effects. It is best used as a decoction or tincture.

PARTS USED: root

MEDICINAL USES: mild laxative, nutritious, anti-inflammatory

SAFETY CONSIDERATIONS: Use with caution if you have a history of kidney stones (due to the oxalate content).

REMEDIES: Herbal Iron Syrup, Yellow Dock Tincture, Digestive Bitters, Gentle Liver Detox Formula, Psoriasis Relief Tea

Sources

A Modern Herbal Volume I, A-H, M. Grieve

A Modern Herbal Volume II, I-Z and Indexes, M. Grieve

Clinical Botanical Medicine, Eric Yarnell, Kathy Abascal, Carol G. Hooper

Herb Contraindications & Drug Interaction, Francis Brinker, N.D.

Herbal Medicine from the Heart of the Earth, Dr. Sharol Marie Tilgner

Nutritional Herbology, Mark Pedersen

The Energetics of Western Herbs, Peter Holmes

The Way of Ayurvedic Herbs, Karta Purkh Singh Khalsa and Michael Tierra

Under the Bramble Arch, Corinne Boyer

Under the Witching Tree, Corinne Boyer

Wild Rose and Western Red Cedar: The Gifts of the Northwest Plants, Elise Krohn

Index

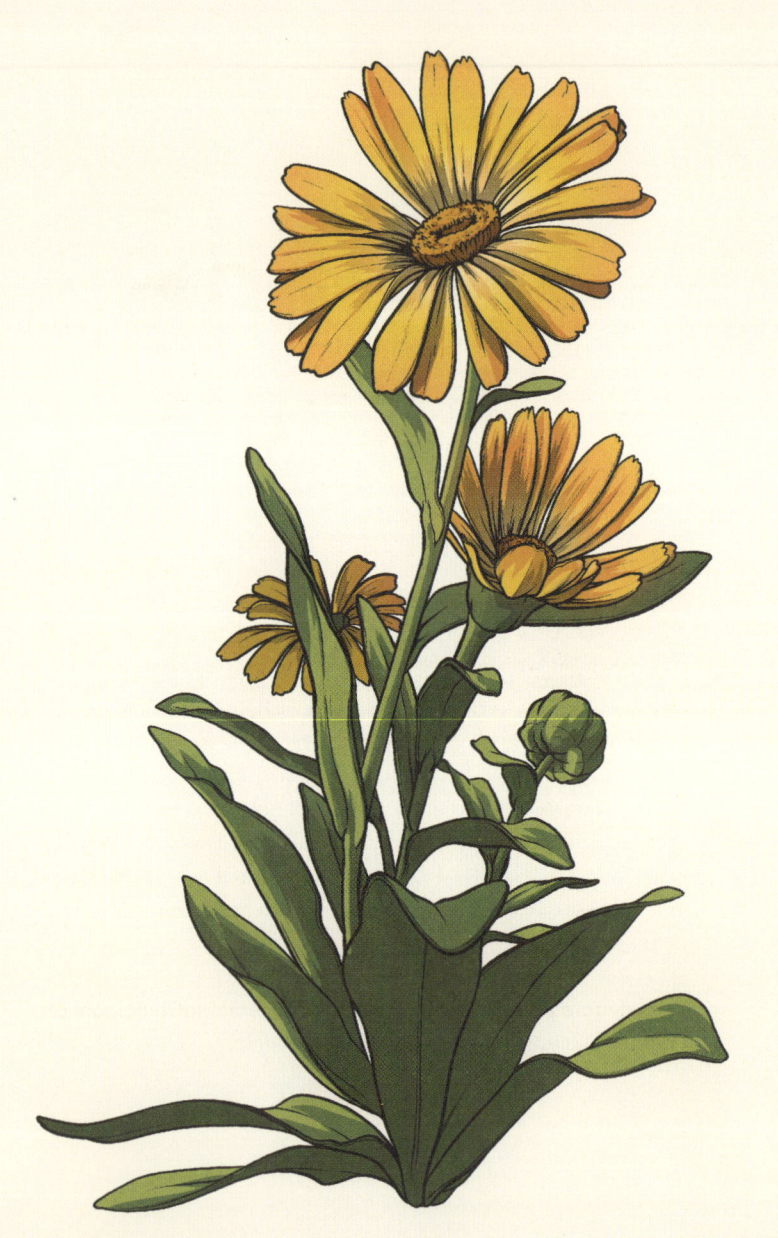

About the Author

ANGELA RENZETTI, LAc, EAMP, RH, is an acupuncturist, herbalist, and teacher with a private practice called Moonlight Medicine in Seattle, Washington. Her work is rooted in Traditional Chinese Medicine, plant medicines, and folk magic. Before becoming an acupuncturist, she lived in China, worked as a translator, and also sang in a band. When she is not treating patients or working with herbs, she is reading, cooking, or going on adventures with her partner. This is her first book.

Learn more about Angela at MoonlightMedicineClinic.com or on social media @moonlightmedicineclinic.

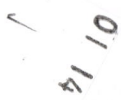

Printed in Colombia

SASQUATCH BOOKS with colophon is a registered
trademark of Blue Star Press, LLC

29 28 27 26 25   9 8 7 6 5 4 3 2 1

The authorized representative in the EU for product safety
and compliance is Authorised Rep Compliance Ltd., Ground
Floor, 71 Lower Baggot Street, Dublin D02 P593, Ireland.
www.arccompliance.com

Text: Angela Renzetti
Editor: Jill Saginario
Production editor: Peggy Gannon
Designer: Anna Goldstein
Illlustrations: Amanda Key

Library of Congress Cataloging-in-Publication
Data is available

ISBN: 978-1-63217-599-1

Sasquatch Books
1325 Fourth Avenue, Suite 1025
Seattle, WA 98101

SasquatchBooks.com

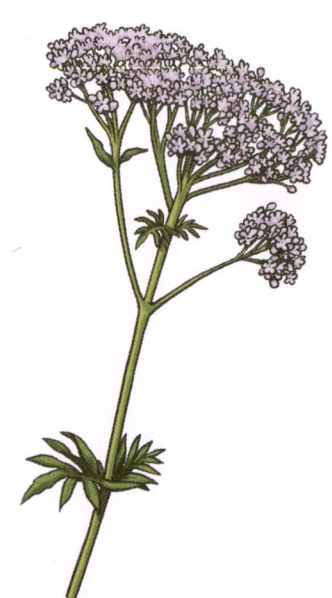